T0114506

Susanna Kaysen

THE CAMERA
MY MOTHER
GAVE ME

Susanna Kaysen is the author of the novels *Far Afield*
and *Asa, As I Knew Him* and the memoir *Girl, Interrupted*.
She lives in Cambridge, Massachusetts.

THE CAMERA
MY MOTHER
GAVE ME

THE CAMERA
MY MOTHER
GAVE ME

· *Susanna Kaysen* ·

VINTAGE BOOKS

A Division of Random House, Inc.

New York

FIRST VINTAGE BOOKS EDITION, OCTOBER 2002

Copyright © 2001 by Susanna Kaysen

The Library of Congress has cataloged the Knopf
edition as follows:
Kaysen, Susanna.
The camera my mother gave me / Susanna Kaysen.—1st ed.
p. cm.
ISBN 0-679-44390-8
I. Title.
2001093864

Vintage ISBN: 978-0-679-76343-7

www.vintagebooks.com

146119709

In memory of my mother,
Annette Neutra Kaysen

THE CAMERA
MY MOTHER
GAVE ME

If you have a vagina you know that most of the time it is without sensation. How does your spleen feel? How do your kidneys feel? How does your pancreas feel? Luckily, we have no idea how these things feel. The vagina is mostly like a pancreas and feels nothing. If it feels something, it is either erotically engaged or ill.

All this is obvious if you have one. But half of us don't.

I have one, and something went wrong with it.

Some days my vagina felt as if somebody had put a cheese grater in it and scraped. Some days it felt as if someone had poured ammonia inside it. Some days it felt as if a little dentist was drilling a little hole in it. The strangest thing was that all these sensations occurred in one inch-long part on the left side. The rest of it was fine.

Gynecology: Fungus

It's a yeast infection, said my gynecologist in June.

On one side? I asked.

I guess it's localized, he said. Here, try this.

This was some antifungal cream. It didn't work.

Hmm, he said, when I returned after a week. Try this.

This was a three-day course of medication in a little bullet that I popped into a plunger and inserted nightly. It didn't work.

There's a stronger version, he said. Let's try that.

That was a cream in a tube. I filled a new plunger with cream and plunged it in. My vagina didn't like that. It became bright red and swollen and hurt worse for four days.

Let's try the pill form, said my gynecologist.

I popped the pill. It made me queasy for two days, but it didn't hurt my vagina.

Now let's do a culture, he said. He emerged from his lab grinning. Not a trace of yeast.

Why does it still hurt? I asked. And why are there red spots here and here? I pointed to the two red spots, one under my clitoris and one on my inner lip. They hurt particularly, I said.

Irritation, he said. Let's try estrogen cream. Use it for ten days. It increases the blood supply and will help it heal.

Estrogen cream dribbled out of me all day long, but for about a week my vagina returned to normal—I didn't feel it. Then it began to twitch and zing again.

That can happen, said my gynecologist.

What?

The estrogen cream causes a yeast infection.

Oh no! I said. Now I'm back where I started.

You're not meant to use it every day, he explained. Twice a week—but I thought it might clear things up.

It did, for a while, I told him.

Let's treat the yeast infection and see where we are.

I went back to the bullet in the plunger.

I like my gynecologist. He is a robust gentleman of Italian origin with a resonant voice and large soft hands. His waiting room used to be decorated with pictures of babies he'd delivered. These days it's decorated with booklets about menopause. Malpractice insurance for obstetricians is very high, I guess.

I met my gynecologist twenty years ago when I had a

cyst in one of the glands in my vagina. That was when I found out how lousy a vagina could feel. He removed this cyst in an operation called a marsupialization—because it makes a little pouch in the vaginal wall where the duct of the gland opens. That way, the gland can't get blocked again.

You know, I said to him after the bullet in the plunger hadn't worked for the second time, it hurts in the same spot as the Bump, or close to it.

One of the good things about having a doctor for twenty years is that you make a language together. "The Bump" is what we call that cyst he removed. Also, after twenty years I'm used to having conversations with him over the top of a sheet while he's got his head between my legs.

In a way, I continued, it feels as if the Bump has returned. It's phantom Bump!

The Bump can't return, he said. But I see what you mean. It's inflamed there. Those red spots are gone, though.

Now what? I asked.

Let's not treat the yeast infection. It'll resolve on its own, usually. Use the estrogen cream twice a week. It will help clear the inflammation, and it increases lubrication. Maybe some of this has to do with less lubrication.

But there isn't less, I said. It's just the same. And wasn't my estrogen level normal?

It was, he said. Three months ago it was.

Sometimes it hurts when I have sex, I said. That's what worries me. You can get a psychological problem from that—associating sex and pain.

Use estrogen, he repeated. And don't avoid sex. You know—he leaned over confidentially—they have shown that the more you use the vagina, the better its health.

My gynecologist had told me this before. That's another thing I like about him. He's very much in favor of sex. So am I, except when it hurts.

I went home with my estrogen cream and my resolve to have sex and maintain vaginal health.

But my vaginal health was declining.

New bad things started to happen. Sharp lines of zinging pain, like a toothache, began to radiate from my former Bump site to the edge of my outer lip, culminating in a dot of soreness. Two things made this worse: driving a car and wearing pants. Then in September, the red spots returned. I went back to the gynecologist.

It's cancer, I told him.

No it isn't, he said. He scraped a bit of skin off and went into his lab. It's not cancer, he repeated when he came out.

Is it herpes? It doesn't feel like herpes.

It's not herpes.

How do you know it's not cancer? I asked.

Cancer doesn't come and go, he said. Cancer just gets worse.

So what is it? I asked him.

I don't know, he said.

Listen, I said, everything's getting worse. I'm really having trouble with sex. My vagina hurts all the time now. If I have sex it hurts more, but it never *doesn't* hurt.

I know, said my gynecologist, but I don't know why. He walked over to the window and looked out. Western medicine doesn't know everything, he said. He turned back to me. I think maybe you should go to an alternative health center.

I was astonished. He was sending me to an herbalist!

There's a very good one here, he went on. They're not cranks. They're real doctors—I know some of them. They specialize in women's health. They aren't going to wave crystals over you or something. I think you ought to try them.

He was washing his hands of me! After twenty years.

But what is it? I asked him. What's wrong with me?

I don't know, he said. Try the alternative health place. The mind and the body—he wiggled his hands around. You have no bacterial infection. You have no fungus. You have no herpes. You have no cancer. I can't tell you why this is happening, but maybe they can.

Independent Study

Here are the things I put into my vagina over the next two months: vinegar rinses; saltwater soaks; a jelly formulated with the correct vaginal pH; and estrogen cream. I tried a lubricant named Astroglide that was more glue than glide. My boyfriend and I tried all sorts of varieties of sexual activity: very quickly, so it wouldn't have time to hurt; without moving, just in there; only fingers in there; nothing at all in there, only outside. Whatever we did, it hurt. I stopped wearing trousers and I drove less. I stood in the health section of the bookstore in Harvard Square and scared myself by reading about vulvar cancer. I spent a lot of time sitting on the floor of the bathroom with a mirror and a flashlight looking at my red spots.

The last activity was interesting. I felt I was doing something forbidden. I would have preferred to look at my vagina in a brighter room, like my study, but I was afraid people would see me doing it (my street is narrow and my neighbors are very close), so I stayed in the dark, shaded bathroom. I felt I wasn't supposed to be investigating it at this length—or at any length, really. But I did. I peered and poked and spread my outer lips and my inner lips and looked into the tunnel of it and tried to figure out what was normal and what wasn't. I had no idea, of course. The more I did it, though, the more I got to know my vagina. And since it was sore in a particular spot, I could compare the rest of it to that spot. I had a control area and a sick area. The trouble was, aside from a little redness, there wasn't much difference between them.

I tried explaining what it felt like to my boyfriend. There's a firecracker in there, I said. It's like a sore throat—I thought this was a helpful image. It's similar to a throat anyhow, so this is a really sore throat. So sore you don't want to swallow, you know that kind of sore throat?

He looked at me quizzically as I made all these analogies.

I don't have one, he said, so I really can't imagine.

You have a throat, I pointed out.

I'm trying to imagine, he said.

We were completely miserable.

My boyfriend was a carpenter. We met because I needed a new front door. My old door had warped and didn't close right. When it snowed, I'd get a small snowdrift in the hall.

He'd fixed that. Curls and chips of fresh wood from the shims for the new door lay at his feet when he was done.

You got a broom? he asked.

I gave him one.

He was careful cleaning up. He made sure to get all the sawdust out of the corners, kneeling down with the dust-pan—You got a dustpan?—and then holding the shavings in place as he walked them to the trash can in the kitchen.

There was something compelling about his slow, thorough care. I decided I needed some bookshelves.

I liked watching him work. I liked his soft-lead pencil shaped like a miniature plank of wood and his spring-loaded yellow tape measure as big as a baseball that hung on his belt and his habit of saying, Okay, here we go, to each piece of lumber before he cut into it.

I especially liked the way he smelled. When I stood beside him while he explained what was going to happen next with the bookshelves, I'd smell the sweetness of cut wood with its bright tang of resin.

Because he was a slow, methodical carpenter I thought he would be a slow, methodical lover too, but he wasn't. He was as energetic and inventive as a jigsaw.

For two years we were happy with the activities we shared: thinking up home improvements for him to make and having sex. Now that I did not want to have sex, though, we got into trouble.

I didn't want to have sex because it hurt. He still did,

which made sense. It didn't hurt him when we had sex. And my vagina still worked in the usual way—if he kissed me, it became soft and approachable and delighted, as if there was nothing wrong with it. But the moment he touched it, I yelped.

We started having a lot of stupid arguments: what video to rent, whether to invite Paula and Ettore for dinner, whether to walk or drive to Harvard Square. These arguments were really about my vagina, and they made it hurt more.

In November I called the alternative health center for an appointment.

Alternative Health

The alternative health center sent me an elaborate questionnaire. What did I eat every day? What herbs and vitamins did I take on a regular basis? What kind of detergent did I use? Was I seeing an acupuncturist or "healer" of any sort? It also asked for a detailed gynecological history, which reassured me somewhat. Along with the questionnaire came a sheet of instructions about what not to do before coming to the center: Don't use perfume, don't use moisturizer or cosmetics, don't smoke. Why? "Some of our patients are allergic."

The alternative nurse was a surprise. She was elegant and elegantly dressed, with understated jewelry and an efficient, attentive manner. I'd been expecting a more Birkenstockian person. She took a long history, did a thorough examination, and then ushered me back into her office for the assessment.

Postsurgical, postherpetic pain syndrome, she said.

The surgery was twenty years ago, I said. And I'm not sure that was herpes. My gynecologist didn't think so.

You've also got an overgrowth of lactobacillus. Do you eat yogurt?

Every day, I said. I put it in there too.

Don't, she said. It's part of the normal flora but you've got too much. That can cause stinging. And maybe you ought to stop eating it for a month or two, just until this settles down. Plus, she said, there's the menopause.

There is no menopause, I said. Everything is the way it always was.

If you're over forty, you're perimenopausal, she said. Then, she went on, there are all those topical antifungals you were taking. They're very irritating to the mucous membranes. Here's what I want you to do. No yogurt, baking soda baths to change the pH, use lubricant during sex—

I tried that, I interrupted her. It doesn't help because I don't need it. I'm lubricated. But I don't want to have sex.

Just try all that, she said, and come back in a month.

The normal pH of the vagina is between 3.8 and 4.2. It's an acidic environment down there. The acidity protects the vagina from bad organisms and promotes good organisms. An upset vagina's pH shifts upward, toward alkalinity. Surgery can provoke this shift, and so can local infections and systemic antibiotics, which kill the good organisms along with the bad and get everything out of whack. And of course menopause does it too. The pH creeps up, making the vaginal environment less efficient at keeping the bothersome things at bay. Then they multiply and dance about and make the tissues sting and sizzle and itch and burn.

Baking soda is alkaline. It took only one baking soda bath for this fact to become vaginally evident. Baking soda made everything worse. I wanted to be a compliant patient, though, so every evening I took my baking soda bath, and every evening my vagina's song of pain got louder and louder. I lay in bed at night with my legs apart trying to air out my crotch and make the stinging subside.

I called the alternative nurse.

Try tea, she said. Soak ten tea bags in a basin of hot water and sit in it for ten minutes after it's cooled down.

All I got from tea was a brown bottom and more stinging. Plus, the tea concoction felt a bit too alternative. I spent fifteen minutes every evening brewing up my basin of tea, then placing it in the bathtub and sloshing into it, spilling the contents, staining the tub and then the towel. I didn't understand why my vagina still hurt, though, because tea is acidic.

I called the alternative nurse again.

Here's what I want you to do, she said. Go to a health-food store and get some empty capsules made of vegetable fiber. Then get some boric acid—

Boric acid! I said. Boric acid?

—fill a capsule with it, and insert it into your vagina every night.

Boric acid kills roaches, I said.

You're a lot bigger than a roach, she said. It won't kill you.

Drugstores don't sell boric acid anymore, because too many people have hurt their eyes or been poisoned from it. I had to go to a hardware store to get it. The box was covered with warnings. Don't ingest! Don't get in eye! If it comes in contact with skin, flush with water! Don't use on mucous membranes!

I decided to heed the warnings and not put it on my mucous membranes.

My alternatives, from alternative health, were limited. I could use the painful and mysterious baking soda—why, if my vagina was insufficiently acidic, was I supposed to make it less acidic? I could use the painful and labor-intensive tea. Or I could use the poisonous boric acid.

I made an appointment with my internist.

Internal Medicine

Before my mother died, I didn't pay much attention to my internist. I didn't like him, but I almost never needed to see him. His specialty was cardiology, and he always wanted to do an electrocardiogram on me even though I was under forty and thin as a rail. Once I smashed my fingernail badly, and when I went to see him, he explained that the only thing to do was heat a needle and then melt a hole in the nail so the blood could come out. But now it's too late, he added. So, shall we do an electrocardiogram?

I didn't really consider him my doctor. But the real one, Doctor Lou, was dead. Heart trouble—that's how I ended up with this guy; he'd been Lou's internist. Lou had been a real doctor: erudite, full of explanations and questions, cautious with his interventions.

But he was dead. And my mother was dead. Watching

my mother die had made me realize that it's important to have a doctor you like. She did. He couldn't stop her from dying, but he didn't leave her to die by herself. I asked if I could be his patient, but for bureaucratic reasons I couldn't. He sent me to Doctor Matthew.

When we met, Doctor Matthew asked me what I wanted from my internist.

Explanations, I said. And somebody who will be with me when I die. Also, no more electrocardiograms!

Sounds reasonable, he said. Then he asked, Weren't you a patient of Lou's?

Yes, I said. Now he's dead.

He was a *real* doctor, said Doctor Matthew.

That clinched it. Okay, I said, You're my doctor now.

I never asked for my record from the other guy. After all, it was just a smashed fingernail, a couple of colds, and half a dozen electrocardiograms.

Nothing of importance had happened to me in the six years I'd been Doctor Matthew's patient, either. But now I had my vaginal story to tell him. By the time I got to the tea episode, he was rolling his eyes.

I'd better take a look at this too, he said. Is that okay?

He'd never needed to do any gynecological things for me because I had my wonderful Italian gynecologist, so this was a novelty—a couple of unexplored inches. I was a little shy, but I wanted his opinion.

Go ahead, I said.

Lots of scar tissue here, he said. Look at this! He was poking around, making me rather uncomfortable.

That hurts, I said.

I'm sure it does, he said. It's all lumps.

But it's been all lumps for twenty years, I said. I had that operation twenty years ago, and it didn't hurt until now.

Menopause, said Doctor Matthew.

I'm tired of hearing about that menopause because it isn't happening, I said.

It's coming, he said.

What do you think of those red spots? I asked.

He poked. Did Tony biopsy those?

Tony is my Italian gynecologist. He scraped them, I said. Normal.

Some kind of inflammation, though. Doctor Matthew emerged from the sheet. Look, he said, scar tissue is inelastic, and also it can't fill with blood like the rest of the vaginal wall, so you've got this lumpy, hard thing, then you've got friction. I think this is basically a mechanical problem. Plus thinning of the tissues from menopause—not that you're having menopause. He laughed. But I really think this might be mechanical.

So now what? I asked. Cortisone? I'd pulled cortisone out of a hat, but he liked it.

Maybe. Sometimes, cortisone can melt scar tissue. You can inject it in there and soften things up.

Great, I said. Will you do that, please?

No way, said Doctor Matthew. I've done it, but in a leg or something. Into the vulva? Forget it. Go back to Tony.

He sent me to alternative health! I protested.

Go back. Explain that I think it's mechanical. Ask him about cortisone. If he doesn't do it, he'll know somebody who does.

But why does it hurt all the time? I asked. Why does it hurt when I'm not having sex? When I'm sitting on the sofa?

I don't know, said Doctor Matthew.

Then I cried for a while. This is horrible, I told him. This is the most horrible thing because it involves someone else too.

Yes, said Doctor Matthew.

It comforted me that he didn't tell me it wasn't the most horrible thing. Whatever is happening to you is always the most horrible thing.

What would help? he asked me.

Never to have sex again, I said.

That's not right for you, he said. Go back to Tony.

Gynecology: Vestibulitis

I've been thinking about you, said Doctor Tony.

It was January, and I was lying on his table again, where I had not been since October. You have? I said. I was surprised.

I think you have something called vestibulitis, he said. The vestibule is the entrance to the vagina. I think you should go see this vulvologist at the Mass. General. The vulva is all he thinks about.

Doctor Matthew thinks it's a mechanical problem having to do with scar tissue from the Bump, I said. He thinks you, or somebody, might try injecting cortisone into it.

Go see the vulvologist, he said. He's a surgeon. He fixes this stuff.

You're a surgeon too, I said. Why go to him?

He can revise the scar. This is his thing, the vulva.

Revise? What does that mean, revise?

Go in there, like underneath the scar, and maybe sever a nerve. You see, the scar tissue can be pressing on a nerve and causing these peculiar sensations—burning, tingling, pain.

Sever a nerve! How does he know which nerve?

Probably he'll use some novocaine and track the nerve. Don't worry. This is all he does.

My gynecologist was standing about four feet away from me with his arms crossed. I did not feel comforted by him.

Listen, I said, sever a nerve! I mean, this is major.

He uncrossed his arms and came a bit closer. I know, he said. There would be a loss of sensation, but he can make it as small as possible. And then this would stop. He leaned closer still. You don't have to live like this. It's been going on for more than six months, right? Go see this guy. And let me know what he says.

Vulvology

How are you getting there? Paula asked.

On the subway, I said.

Forget that, she said. I'm taking you.

We were sitting in her kitchen. Some veal stew was simmering on the stove, clouding the windows. It was February, and cold. Ettore was in the front room, painting and listening to Coltrane play "In a Sentimental Mood."

It's at the Mass. General, I said. There isn't anywhere to park down there.

They have a parking lot, said Paula. You have no idea what he's going to do to you.

Well, he isn't going to do it *then*, I said.

Track the nerve? Isn't that what you said? Paula wriggled her shoulders. Eeeee, she said.

Okay, okay, I said. The appointment's tomorrow at two.

Ettore came in. What appointment?

Hers, said Paula. Nothing for you.

Where's that yellow pigment I got yesterday? he asked. He opened the refrigerator and closed it again.

You left it in the hall, said Paula. Are you hungry?

I don't know, he said. He sat down at the table with us. Anything new? he asked me.

Nothing good, I said. What are you working on?

Tiger maple.

We have some nice new clients with a mansion in the Back Bay, said Paula. Rich Russians.

I didn't know there were any rich Russians, I said.

Ettore laughed. These might be the only two, he said. They want a tiger maple mantelpiece.

Nobody ever had such a thing, I objected.

I told them that, he said. I told them I could make a nice yellowish marble, that would be correct for the *palazzo*. He shrugged. They want what they want.

Paula said, They want the sample by Monday.

I'm doing it, said Ettore. Relax.

Isn't tiger maple for furniture? I asked.

Usually. Ettore tapped his fingers with Coltrane. For a desk maybe, or a bureau. We don't even have it in Italy.

No maples? I asked.

We got maples, he said. But not like here. Not a million maples. He stood up. Okay, he said. He tapped on my head a few times. Still *la passera*? he asked.

La passera means "the sparrow." It's an Italian endearment for the vagina.

Yup, I said. The perpetual *passera.*

Judging from the vulvologist's waiting room, a lot of women in the greater Boston area had sore vaginas. Paula and I sat together leafing through *Family Circle* magazine and discussing in a nervous sort of way whether afterward we would go down Charles Street to look at antiques. I couldn't imagine "afterward" because I couldn't imagine what was going to happen when I got into the examining room. I kept having an image of a dentist's novocaine needle—enormous and sheathed in a stainless-steel carapace—heading into my vagina.

The examining room was the size of a broom closet and had no window. I waited in there another twenty minutes.

When the vulvologist came in I was struck by how much his face resembled a vulva. He had soft, mushy features and a little wispy mustache. He fired off a lot of questions.

Did your gynecologist give you cortisone? Did your gynecologist give you estrogen cream? Did your gynecologist treat you for a yeast infection? Does it hurt when you drive?

It always hurts, I told him.

Okay, he said. He sounded pleased. I'll be back in a minute.

Then the nurse came in and told me to get on the table.

The vulvologist came back and settled down on a stool between my legs.

Here, I said, pulling open my vagina and pointing to the sore spots, is where it hurts. I was an old hand at this, after Doctor Tony, Doctor Matthew, the alternative nurse, and my hours with the mirror.

Well, that's not where the problem is, said the vulvologist. He slid in the speculum. Then he picked a Q-Tip off a tray, and all of a sudden I felt a really remarkable pain, the sort you gasp from. I gasped.

That's where the problem is, he said.

Wow, was all I could say.

How many times did you have surgery on this Bartholin's gland?

Once, I said. I didn't know you could do it more than that.

Oh yeah, said the vulvologist. He continued to elicit astonishing pain from somewhere inside me with his Q-Tip.

I writhed around a bit on the table.

All right, he said. I'm going to track this. He began to prod all over my inside. Does this hurt? Does this hurt? Does this hurt?

Luckily, none of it hurt.

Does this hurt?

Wow, I said. It hurt.

This went on for about five minutes.

Give me the mirror, he said to the nurse. Sit up, he told me.

I propped myself up on my elbows. It's not easy to sit up when you're lying on a hard examining table with your legs spread, and there's a speculum inside you and a vulva-faced doctor sitting with his nose in your crotch.

Look here, he said. He pulled at my sore lips. See this? He pointed with his abominable Q-Tip at the dimple Doctor Tony had made in my vaginal wall twenty years before. See the way it's red around the opening? That's where the problem is.

Why does it hurt farther out? I asked.

Now we're going to try the novocaine, he said. He ducked down between my legs and fiddled around with something. It'll be cold, he said.

I braced myself. But it was just cold.

It's a liquid, the nurse told me, not a shot. I relaxed a little.

I'll be back, said the vulvologist.

It might sting, said the nurse. Then she left too.

It stung.

After about five minutes, he returned.

Why did this happen? I asked him.

Eh, he said. He shrugged.

What is it, anyhow?

Eh, he said. He returned to the stool and resumed his Q-Tip.

Does this hurt? Does this hurt? Does this hurt?

It hurts a little, I said.

Not like before, he told me. Before, you were jumping off the table. Good, now we know that novocaine works. He turned to the nurse. Bring me the dilators, he said.

I didn't bother to ask any more questions while we waited.

The nurse came back with a bunch of thick glass sticks.

What are you going to do with those? I asked. I felt alarmed.

The vulvologist picked one up and handed it to me. It was heavy. Put that in, he said.

Oh, it's a dildo, I said. I put it in.

Does that hurt? he asked.

It hurts a little.

Okay, he said. Now try this one.

This one was bigger. It hurt more. I told him so.

But it goes in, he said.

I guess it does, I admitted.

Now this one. He handed me something about the size of a baseball bat.

That's too big, I said.

Put it in.

I put it in. It felt really nasty.

See, it went in, he said. Okay. He handed me another.

I can't— I started to say.

Put it in, he said.

It went in fine. That didn't hurt, I said.

For the first time, something animated crossed the vulvologist's face. It remembers! he crowed. That was the second one, which you said hurt. Now it doesn't hurt. See? It stretches, and it remembers.

Okay, I said. I wasn't as excited about it as he was.

He handed me a plastic version of the medium-sized dildo.

Use this, he said. It will remember. Put the novocaine in before intercourse and you'll be functional. He stood up. Some people never come back, he said. He sat down again. You have to put the novocaine right on that spot I showed you, and nowhere else. It's very strong. But then, you'll be functional. He stood up and pushed his stool against the wall. The nurse left the room carrying all the dildos.

What's the matter with me? I asked.

You have a sore spot, he said. Then, rather offhandedly, he added, I could cut it out.

Cut it out?

Yup.

And does that work?

Yup.

And what is the problem? I asked again.

Some people think it's a disorder of the pelvic-floor muscles, he said. Some people think it has to do with oxylates in the urine irritating the vulva. There are people upstairs who work on the pelvic-floor muscles. You could try that.

Does that work? I asked him.

Eh, he said. Some people use tricyclic antidepressants to minimize the pain.

Does that work?

Eh.

I felt stymied. This operation, what kind of operation is it?

Day surgery, said the vulvologist.

That didn't tell me much. They'd say that about open-heart surgery these days. I tried again.

Is it comparable to the Bartholin's cyst removal?

Um, he said. Uh.

I took that for a yes.

Some people never come back, he repeated. I'll give you a prescription for novocaine and another numbing agent that isn't as strong. You can try those. Come back if you want surgery.

I got dressed and went out to the waiting room, where Paula was reading *Family Circle* for the twentieth time.

Let's go to Marika, I said.

The Agate Bowl

Marika is an old fixture on Charles Street that specializes in porcelain and jewelry. It is dim and thick with dust and completely enclosed in security iron and always looks shut. It was open, though. Paula and I stood at the jewelry counter and asked to see all the trays: the small earring tray, the cameo tray, the pearl necklace tray and the broken pearl necklace tray, which is separate and usually less expensive, the coral tray, the amber, the lapis, the African trading beads. The woman behind the counter brought each tray out alone and put it beside a swatch of black velvet on the glass. She tucked the tray back into its spot below the counter before bringing out the next.

We became interested in coral. We tried on many coral necklaces. I was particularly taken by a dark, two-stranded one, slightly bigger than a choker and the color of raw salmon.

You should get that, said Paula. You have to get a nice thing after that appointment.

I don't know if I'd wear it, I said. Is it too strange, with these lumps? It was the unfinished sort of coral, not worked into beads. It looked a bit savage.

Get it, said Paula, and then you'll wear it. Paula is practical.

She'd found a good one too. It was the pale, pearly color, which is better for her because she is fair and has a spattering of fair freckles.

You should get that, I said.

I didn't have a horrible appointment, she said.

For a minute we stood looking at each other wearing coral necklaces we weren't going to buy. Then we took them off and put them back in the tray.

I looked up at the shelf behind the counter, where an assortment of carved figurines and stopped gold clocks and silver objects stood in a pile of dust. What's that green thing? I asked the woman.

This green thing? She picked up a Japanese jade squirrel, hideous.

No, no, I said. That bowl thing to the left.

Oh, that. She brought it to me. It's a Chinese bowl. It's agate.

It was about four inches across, with a slightly flared rim and a small ridge on the bottom, carved from a piece of agate the color of pea soup and shot through with black flecks and stripes. I held it up. Even in Marika's dim light I could see my fingers through the stone.

Is it old? I asked.

Yeah, said the woman. Yeah, it's pretty old.

This is what I want, I said. I leaned over to Paula. It's my vagina, I whispered, that bowl.

It was very expensive, and I bought it.

As we walked back up Charles Street to the parking garage, my vagina began to throb and sting. The novocaine was wearing off. When we got into her car, I had trouble sitting down. I couldn't find a position that didn't feel bad. Keeping my butt off the seat helped, so I braced myself between my back and my legs, which I pressed on the dashboard. But that hurt my back, so I sank down onto the seat and throbbed.

Hurts, huh? Paula said.

It does, I said.

Glad I came? she asked.

I nodded. The pain was getting worse by the minute.

I don't think I could have done this without you, I said. I mean, I couldn't walk if I had to walk right now.

There you go, said Paula.

Numb

It took several days to recover from the vulvologist's activities, and then I was ready to try novocaine cream. I'd decided to try it by myself. I didn't want my boyfriend and his attentions confusing my experiment.

According to the patient insert, novocaine cream is used mostly in the mouth. There were a lot of warnings about biting the tongue, inability to swallow, and choking. It's good for intubating people—you can smear it all along the tube before you stick it down somebody's throat or windpipe. I didn't want to think about that.

I sat on the floor of the bathroom with my mirror and attempted to put a dab of novocaine cream on the precise spot the vulvologist had shown me. Two things made this difficult: The spot was so far inside that I had to hold my vagina open with one hand to reach it; and the novocaine cream tended to melt off my finger before I could put it anywhere. On the third try I got some to stick in there. Then I went downstairs to the sofa to await the numbing.

Within about three minutes I felt an intense pain in my vagina. I began to sweat. Before the novocaine cream—in the minutes just before I put it in—my vagina had been at its usual zingy level, a continuo of simmering irritation that I had learned, over the previous eight months, to live with. This new feeling was not livable with. Probably because I was worn out from all the things that had happened to my vagina at the vulvologist's office, I felt really scared. I had the terrible thought: It will always feel like this and I can't stand it.

The pain went away though, and I felt a sort of numbness, eventually. It wasn't a thorough or pleasant numbness. It was like the tail end of a novocaine shot, when you're standing on the bus after the dentist appointment and your tongue and gums are starting to come back: a sort of half-dead sensation. That lasted for three-quarters of an hour. Then my vagina went back to slightly worse than normal, zinging and stinging in its everyday way.

My boyfriend had high hopes for the novocaine cream, especially after I'd reported the vulvologist's claim that I would be "functional" with it.

Did you try it? he asked when he got home.

Um, I said.

And?

It's bad. It hurts really bad.

But do you get numb?

Kind of numb, I said. But I don't think it's worth it.

Let's fuck, he said.

No, I said. Now it's not numb.

Put some more in! He was eager to try.

No, I said. I don't want to put any more in ever.

Then we were mad at each other again.

I made an appointment with Doctor Matthew. I made one with my Italian gynecologist too, just in case.

Professional Ethics

That could be from alcohol, Doctor Matthew said. He left the examining room and came back with a huge drug book. Yeah, he continued, that's formulated with alcohol. That would hurt like hell on irritated tissue. Here's one in a different base. Not as strong, only two percent novocaine instead of five. But it's worth a try. I'll give you a prescription for that.

Listen, I said, the whole visit was very upsetting. I didn't get any information at all.

Surgeons? suggested Doctor Matthew.

All he said was, I could cut that out.

I'm sure he could. Doctor Matthew smiled. You probably ought to find out more about it.

I'll say, I said, but I won't find it out from him. I think I'll go to Doctor Tony and see what he knows about this operation.

That's an excellent idea, said Doctor Matthew.

Doctor Tony had a different theory about the novo-caine cream.

That reaction ought to stop, he said. That's a reaction to the numbing agent. It's also part of the treatment.

You mean it's supposed to hurt?

It zaps the nerves. Jangles them.

To confuse them? I was mystified.

Exactly, said Doctor Tony. It jangles them out of their usual pathways. Some people are treating this problem with red-pepper extract.

Oh my God! I said. I had to cross my legs just thinking of it.

Wild, huh? said Doctor Tony. What I think you should do is use it every day for a few weeks and see if the reaction stops and also if the general sensations die down. They might, you know.

A few weeks! It really, really hurts, I said.

And if it doesn't help, he went on, I think you'll have to have the operation.

I hated this man, I confessed.

He's absolutely the best.

He wouldn't tell me a thing. Nothing.

Surgeons, Doctor Tony explained. Also, the Mass. General.

What about it?

He was reluctant to articulate it, but he tipped his head

this way and that, indicating a bothersome situation. You know, he said, it's the Mass. General and all that.

I got it. Maybe he'd tell *you*? I asked.

Maybe. Doctor Tony didn't look hopeful. He might send me a report.

And will you explain it to me?

Of course I will, he said.

Research

Many of my friends went to medical school, but only one is a practicing physician, my next-door neighbor Laura. I started with her.

Don't go under the knife without doing research, she said.

Right, I said. But what kind of research?

Read the articles. She was sitting at her kitchen table with a pile of fabric swatches, trying to pick material for curtains. The dog was at her feet chewing on an exhausted doll. The cat was sitting on the editorial page of *The Boston Globe*. The turtle was asleep in its vat on the windowsill. The children were at school. Scott, Laura's husband, was in his study writing a novel and keeping a distance from Girl Things like curtains and vaginas.

What articles?

These surgeons write articles about what they do, especially when they come up with new procedures. Read them and see what outcomes they get. If you don't understand, bring them to me.

Where am I going to find them?

On the Net, she said. Now, these are the two patterns I'm thinking about. She held them up. One had grape leaves; the other had chrysanthemums.

Don't get patterned curtains, I said. You're going to have so much material—I pointed at the two huge windows—that you'd get sick of any pattern.

Hmm, said Laura. I bet you're right.

For research, you need a research scientist. I called my friend Maria, who is a molecular biologist. She investigates yeast. When she picked up the phone, I could hear her clacking away on the computer in her lab.

Hey Maria, I said, can you do some computer thing for me?

Sure, she said. Then she said, Are you ever going to get a computer? You might like it.

I don't think so, I said. I need to find some articles by this surgeon about the operation he does on the vagina.

Oh darling! Are you going to have that?

I want to read about it first, I said.

You'd better, she told me. I'll find them. Give me his name and the name of the disease, or whatever it is.

Whatever it is, I repeated. Who knows what it is. It's called vestibulitis.

I'll put my research assistant on it too. We should come up with something in a day or so.

Come for dinner when you get it, I said.

Three days later Maria came for dinner. She had a sheaf of paper in one hand and a bunch of daffodils in the other.

Aren't they beautiful? she said. She put her nose in the flowers. And they smell like grass.

What's all that stuff? asked my boyfriend.

Articles about this surgery, I said.

You're not going to understand that, he said.

Laura said she'd help me.

I can help you too, said Maria. But it's only one article, and it's old. It's from 1989. My assistant did a subject search, though, and came up with other things.

Is it bad that it's old? I asked her.

It's kind of peculiar, she said. That's nearly a decade. Hasn't he done anything *new*?

I guess it's different with surgeons, I said. It's not like your things. They aren't always making discoveries.

Maria sniffed. She has the researcher's disdain for the practitioner.

My boyfriend was leafing through the papers. I don't understand this stuff, he said. It's not worth bothering with anyhow. You should just do what he says.

Who? I asked.

That pussy doctor.

No, said Maria. You have to find out more.

Are *you* a doctor? My boyfriend was getting upset.

That's not the point, she said. You have to be a well-informed patient.

You're not going to understand this stuff, he repeated, ignoring her. What's the point of going to a doctor if you don't listen to what he says?

If somebody was going to do an operation on your dick, you'd want to find out if it was absolutely necessary, I said.

I guess so, he admitted.

We ate a chicken roasted with a lot of garlic. Then my boyfriend went out for a walk. I'll let you girls talk, he said.

How can you live with that? asked Maria. Just do what the doctor tells you. What kind of thinking is that?

Hey, I said, lots of people think that way. People much more sophisticated than he is. Anyhow, he has his charms.

She lifted her chin a little to signify that she was not as charmed as I was. I gather he does, she said.

Maria is my only unmarried woman friend, and we have had many detailed discussions of our erotic lives. My married friends are more discreet, or else they have less to discuss.

That's not his only charm, I said. He's emotionally transparent. It's comforting. Whatever he feels, I know it. He can't disguise it.

If that makes you happy— She didn't finish her sentence. Maria believes in romance, probably because she is Polish. On the other hand, because she is also tall and beautiful, she gets a lot of romance, which gives her the impression that it's easy to come by.

Maria had brought a number of abstracts of articles, one by my vulvologist. There was also a ten-page informational booklet about my disease from the National Vulvodynia and Vestibulitis Association. I read this eagerly. It described what I had. It offered the various theories I'd heard from the vulvologist—pelvic-floor muscles, oxylates in the urine—and listed some other theories: allergy to topical medications, to scented toilet paper and soap or tampons; chronic or recurrent yeast infections or herpes outbreaks; some unknown relationship between vulvar pain and chronic bladder infection; an as-yet-unidentified virus. What it added up to was, They didn't know.

I called Maria. Can you get the articles themselves? These are just the abstracts.

Things are a bit crazy here, she said. I have a grant due. If we can't just get them off the Net it might be a while.

If you can, I said.

She called back two days later. Listen, she said, this grant—

Maria always has a grant due. That's how it is with research scientists.

Never mind, I said. I'll ask Jamie.

See, we can't get them off the Net. It's a whole business with interlibrary loan.

It's fine, I said. What you got helps because now I know what to look for. Jamie can get it all from Countway.

Jamie used to be a doctor in occupational health. But he didn't like it. He liked thinking about statistics. So he quit, and now he thinks about statistics in epidemiology. I called him at the School of Public Health.

Sure, he said. Tell me the journals.

I'd narrowed what I wanted down to two articles: one by the vulvologist, published in *Obstetrics and Gynecology*, and one that was an overview of the literature, published in the *Clinical Journal of Pain*. I liked the title *Clinical Journal of Pain*. I could think of a lot of articles to write for them: "Impacted Wisdom Tooth"; "Twisted Ankle in the Subway"; "Inappropriate Boyfriends."

Jamie, however, didn't like the *Clinical Journal of Pain*. Never heard of that, he said. The other one's easy.

He turned up the next afternoon with it. He'd been running, and the article was somewhat damp from being stuffed inside his running jacket.

This is a crazy operation, he said.

It is?

Who is this guy? Hasn't he written anything since 1989?

That's just what Maria said, I told him. I handed him the

booklet from the Vulvodynia Association. Take a look at this, I said.

He sat down on the sofa and took a look at it. Sounds like what you got, he said. They don't recommend the surgery, he added.

I know, I said. But they've got some weird recommendations. Like don't eat lettuce.

That oxylate stuff.

Do you buy that? I asked.

He shrugged. What do I know? I'm not a doctor. Sounds fishy. That *Clinical Journal of Pain*, he went on, I tried to get it out of Countway, and you'll never believe what happened. That volume, *that* volume, is missing!

Missing, huh? I said. I wasn't surprised. This sort of thing always happens to Jamie. What he wants is missing, or he left it in someone's car, or the cleaning woman threw it away. In this case, though, it was what I wanted that was missing.

Thanks for trying, I said. What's so crazy about the operation?

You read it, he said. I wouldn't do it. He zipped up his jacket and ran off down the street.

I read it.

"Patients underwent laser ablation of the area to a depth of 5mm to 1cm. Increasing depth of treatment ceased after the 5-mm point if bleeding was encountered. . . . Among those in whom laser treatment failed . . . we excised an eliptical specimen encompassing the area between the hymenal ring and the perineal body ridge extending to both Bartholin duct apertures."

I got out my ruler and looked at five millimeters and one centimeter. Either amount seemed to be too much to "excise" from the wall of my vagina. I read on.

"Among laser-treated patients, the main complication was a long healing phase of up to ten weeks' duration." Two and a half months with a vagina that was basically an open wound.

"The potential morbidity of excision with perineoplasty can be considerable. Local hemorrhage and hematoma are possible complications in this very vascular area."

When my boyfriend got home that night, I told him I wasn't having the operation.

How come?

It's too horrible. They scrape off about half an inch of the inside, all around. They just scrape it off!

And does it work?

It depends who you listen to. The vulvologist says it works. The people in Michigan who have a center for this disease say it works about half the time.

So it works, he said.

Half the time. Suppose I'm in the other half?

But you can't fuck at all now. Maybe you'll be able to fuck.

This got me mad. But maybe I won't, and I'll have a big bleeding miserable vagina for two months. Or forever—who knows? Maybe it will just go away on its own, I said hopelessly. I'd been saying that for almost a year.

You've been saying that for about a year, said my boyfriend.

I need to get this other article, I said. This other article talks about all the articles that have been written about this disease.

Why do you keep reading these articles you don't understand?

I understand enough to know I don't want to do it.

You're not a doctor, he said.

It's *my* vagina, I said. That vulvologist doesn't have a vagina. If he did, he wouldn't do this to it. And Jamie said he wouldn't have this operation.

He hasn't got a pussy either, said my boyfriend. And he's not a doctor.

He used to be, I said.

Oh, what does he know? said my boyfriend.

The two remaining friends who went to medical school are a couple, both psychoanalysts. They've known me since I was two, and they are an extra set of parents for me. They both grew up in medical families—Sanford in Nebraska, Ingrid in Sweden. I went there for dinner and explained about the *Clinical Journal of Pain* article.

Oh, I can find you that in a jiffy, said Sanford. He loves bibliographic research.

Jamie the epidemiologist said the volume was missing at Countway.

Maybe not, said Sanford. Or maybe it's back now. He has a hopeful disposition. He went down to his basement office to get onto the Harvard Library computer line.

I sat in the kitchen with Ingrid and complained about what a mess my vagina was. It never stops hurting, I said. Like right now, it feels like some jagged thing is sticking up there, poking and scraping.

Pretty bad, she said, shaking her head. That's really lousy. And then you get spasms.

What spasms?

If it hurts, then the muscles get spasms and that just makes it hurt more.

I haven't noticed any spasms, I said.

Sure. Tightens up.

How would I know? I said. I never use it anymore.

You wouldn't want to, said Ingrid, with all that.

Sanford came upstairs shaking his head. I'll have to get it from interlibrary loan, he said. But that won't be a problem. Probably by the end of the week I'll have it.

We ate goulash.

Four days later Ingrid called. We have it, she said. Come for dinner whenever you can.

I'll come tomorrow, I said. I had to give my boyfriend warning when I went out to dinner. We had a deal that I could go to see Sanford and Ingrid once a week. This would be twice in the same week.

They're helping me with the article I want, I explained.

Fucking articles, he said. Then he made a visible effort to be nice. Okay, honey, you go there. You say hi to Sanford.

My boyfriend liked Sanford. When urban renewal came to Boston, Sanford had salvaged a lot of decorative pieces from turn-of-the-century buildings that were being demolished. He'd made friends with the wreckers, and for several weeks had come home with a huge copper finial in the backseat of his car or a fluted mahogany pillar tied onto the roof. He'd then attached these things to his front porch. He'd stuck objects shaped like a bishop's miter or a chef's hat on top of run-of-the-mill four-by-four fence posts and hung immense teak swags off railings three inches wide. After thirty years these arrangements were breaking down. My boyfriend had spent a couple of afternoons helping to shore things up. He'd returned impressed with Sanford. He's got some amazing weird shit there, he told me. Had it all put together with string and Elmer's Glue-All, though.

The next night I walked past the topknots perched at the corners of the porch, the half-moon stained glass hanging off the clapboards on picture wire, the chipped marble something-or-other that served as an outdoor table, and rang the bell at Sanford and Ingrid's house. Inside, the table was set and the article was beside my plate.

What do you think? I asked them.

Pretty bad, said Ingrid.

You'll see when you read it, said Sanford. The main thing is, they postulate it as a pain syndrome.

What does that mean?

Certain sorts of pain lead to anomalies in the central nervous system, in pain perception. Then it becomes a kind of feedback loop. But they don't *know*.

What sorts of pain? I asked. Like in places that don't usually feel pain?

That's one kind, said Sanford. If you stimulate pain in a usually insensate area.

So it's a kind of nerve damage?

Not quite, said Ingrid. That implies direct trauma. It's more that the nerves are misinterpreting, that the central nervous system is saying there's pain but there isn't pain.

Sympathetically maintained pain, it's called, said Sanford.

It was a rather grim dinner.

Oh God, I said, in the middle of peeling a pear, I just don't know what to do next. Maybe I should go back to the alternative nurse.

Biofeedback, Sanford suggested. That's quite successful with this sort of thing.

What is this sort of thing? I asked. I don't get it. Is it like phantom-limb pain?

In the same category, he said. Similar.

Also stress, said Ingrid.

Stress what?

Wouldn't help, she said. It wouldn't help whatever it is.

But it causes stress! I objected.

That's the trouble, she agreed.

When I got home, my boyfriend was asleep, and I stayed up late reading the article. It covered everything I'd heard about, in great detail: oxylates, allergic reactions to antifungal medicine, pelvic-floor muscle spasms, and, its particular focus, sympathetically maintained pain.

One sentence struck me: "There is . . . evidence that inflammation of visceral organs can induce a similar altered sensitivity in the dorsal horn neurons of the spinal cord, a phenomenon referred to as central sensitization. Such changes in central neural function are thought to play a significant role in the development of pathological pain."

I hid the article in my desk drawer. Then I went to bed and dreamed of the neurons in my dorsal horn, which I visualized as a stubby tail, thick and hot with pain, sticking out of my back. In the morning I made an appointment with the alternative nurse.

Alternative Health Two

In November, when I first saw the alternative nurse, I was on a short vacation from regular medicine, exploring the strange customs of a foreign outpost. Now, in March, I was an émigré to this place. The plane had broken down, the boat had sunk, there wasn't any way home.

I want you to keep a pain diary, said the nurse.

My whole life is a pain diary, I said.

Use a scale of zero to five, and make at least two notes a day about your pain level, every day for a month.

Is five the worst pain I've ever felt or the worst my vagina has ever felt?

Oh, the vagina, she said. Let's just keep it all in the family.

And that's it? I asked.

I hate to put you back on baking soda, since it made things worse. Unless you want to try again.

I don't, I said. Then I described the vulvologist and his operation.

She knew all about it. Yup, she said. That's his thing. That's what he has to offer.

Does it work?

Sometimes. It works about forty-five percent of the time.

That isn't much for a surgical procedure, I said. Suppose appendectomies worked less than half the time?

She nodded. Well, you have to think that it does work almost half the time. If you want to do it, that is.

Should I do it?

You'd have to decide that, she said. Now, how about intercourse?

What's intercourse? I said.

She laughed. Then she said, You really have to try. It's bad if you don't.

How can I? I asked. It hurts so much, and then it hurts for days and days afterward, so I don't want to.

How about other kinds of sexual activity?

Nothing is any good, I said. Everything hurts. Anything hurts. Just getting aroused hurts—is that possible?

Sure, she said. More blood, more sensation.

The other problem— I stopped.

Yes? she said.

My boyfriend wants to *fuck*. That's where he wants to

SUSANNA KAYSEN

end up. It's like we can't start and then not go all the way
there.

A lot of men are like that, she said. She grinned. You
can't blame them. It feels good.

It used to feel good to me too, I said. That's finished.

You don't know that. She leaned closer to me over her
desk. I've seen people much worse off than you get better.

How? I sounded petulant.

It takes time, she said. Okay, keep the diary, and prom-
ise me you'll try intercourse—or something—a few times.

I might, I said.

· 56 ·

The Home Front

What did the pussy nurse say? asked my boy-friend that night.

She said we should try to fuck.

Great! he said. Let's go try.

I'm making dinner, I said. I knew that was a stupid objec-tion. I could have stopped making dinner. We'd missed plenty of dinners before my vagina got sick.

You just don't want to, he said.

No, I don't, I said. How can I, when it hurts?

If you never do it, you're going to get all out of shape and it's going to hurt for sure.

That's not why, I said. But I felt uneasy, because he was making the same point the alternative nurse had made. My gynecologist had made this point as well. So I said, insis-tently, It hurts because there's something wrong with it.

He scowled. I think you're just looking for an excuse.

I'm *not!* An excuse for what?

What am I supposed to think? Nobody knows what the hell is wrong with it. Maybe there isn't anything wrong with it. What's wrong with it is you don't want to fuck me anymore.

There's only one way to disprove that assertion. And the truth was, I did still want to fuck him, in an abstracted, nostalgic sort of way. That is, if I'd wanted to fuck at all, I would have wanted to fuck him. But I didn't want to.

We went to bed. For a while it was nice—more than nice. It was novel and thrilling, as if we had just met. We hadn't approached each other in more than a month. I was surprised by how wonderful I could feel. I was used to feeling lousy most of the time. The sensations of excitement were overwhelming. I'd forgotten about that. Then he pushed himself into me and it was horrible.

First I felt as if I were being torn or sliced. As he settled into a rhythm, I felt that something was scraping me over and over in the same raw spot, until the rawness and soreness were all I could feel. He didn't notice. He was intent on what he was doing. I decided to let him get on with it, but the pain was really bothering me. I pulled away inside myself, so that the events on the bed were far from where "I" was, and the pain was far away also. That worked, but I didn't like doing it. There was something nasty about it. I had the thought, People who don't like sex must feel this way. Then I realized that now I was somebody who didn't like sex.

My boyfriend dropped his head to my shoulder and kissed my neck. That was so nice, honey, he said. Oh, that was so nice.

Um, I said noncommittally. I was exhausted.

After dinner I made my first entry in my pain diary. I had to decide how to rank my "resting state" on a scale of zero to five. Zero was only a memory. Five was how I'd felt in bed that evening. Two, I decided, was my usual condition.

Day One, I wrote. At normal, level two. After intercourse, five plus.

That night I had trouble sleeping. My vagina was hot, as if it had a fever. I made a tent out of the covers by drawing my knees up; then I arranged an air vent on the side to cool things down. That helped, but it was a hard way to sleep. My tent-and-vent would collapse and then my vagina would overheat and I'd wake up. A few days later, though, I was back at level two.

I was looking forward to sleeping without my tent as I got into bed that night. I curled up on my side and thought about how tired I was.

You asleep? asked my boyfriend.

Mmm, I said. I knew what was going to happen next.

Honey? he said. I felt the weight of his penis on the back of my thigh. Honey?

I can't, I said. It hurts too much.

Does it hurt right now?

It's bearable now. If we fuck, it will hurt.

But you said you'd try!

I tried, I told him.

Once. You tried once.

I didn't say anything. I lay on my side and hated him.

Can't we try again? He'd slid himself between my legs already.

I realized I wanted to hate him. It helped me, because then I could pretend it was all his fault. So I didn't object again. And I stayed up late with my tent, hating him.

Day Four, I wrote the next morning. Before intercourse, level two. After intercourse, five plus plus.

It went on like this for another week. Then I called the alternative nurse.

The Brain

I was sitting on the alternative nurse's examining table draped in a sheet and hugging my legs. I'd been describing the events of the previous week.

Is this some way of turning against him? I asked her. Is this a hysterical illness? He thinks it is.

No, said the alternative nurse. There are physiological changes. I saw them two minutes ago. Red patches and particular areas of sensitivity. Just because we don't understand the cause doesn't mean it isn't real.

What do you mean by real? I asked. Hysterical paralysis is real if you can't move your arm.

But you *could* move your arm. There's nothing wrong with your arm. Something is wrong with your vagina. She put her hand on my drawn-up knees. This is part of what's so bad about this disease. People feel responsible for it.

It gets worse if I'm upset, though, I said. If we start to fight about having sex, my vagina hurts more right away.

Look, she said, stress alters the pH of the vagina. Did you know that?

Yes, I said. I can feel that it does. But that's what worries me. Maybe it's like an ulcer. It's all from stress.

Turns out ulcers aren't from stress, she said. Turns out there's a bacterium. She moved her hand to my shoulder. Listen. I want to try a different approach. I want to get you some relief as soon as possible. I want you to try amitriptyline.

That's an antidepressant, I said.

This is a subclinical dose. In small doses, it seems to affect the fibers that innervate the vulva. It alters the perception of pain.

I'm morally opposed to antidepressants, I said. Then I laughed, because it sounded ridiculous. For myself, I added. You can take one if you want.

I'm talking about a tiny amount, she said. Won't you try? Tiny, tiny.

What's it going to do to me?

It might make your mouth dry. It might make you tired, so take it before bed. And if you feel groggy in the morning, take it a bit earlier, like after dinner.

I don't want to do it, I said.

Will you just try for a month?

A month!

Just try, please, she said. I think it's going to work. We use it for a lot of chronic pain.

I stopped at the pharmacy on the way home from her office.

Over the previous eight months my pharmacist and I had become friendly. I'd been in nearly every week, and each time I had a different prescription: antifungal, antibacterial, hormonal, numbing. At this point, she was trying to spare me some expense.

I don't even want to try this stuff, I told her.

She grinned. You know, she said, you can get just a week's worth if you want. You can fill the rest of the prescription later. In fact, you can get two pills if you want.

I thought it over. Give me three, I said. I'll know after three.

As she handed them over, she said: Dry mouth, drowsiness, upset stomach. Blurry vision sometimes.

Sounds great, I said.

One of the things I liked about her was she'd never asked what was wrong. Maybe she'd figured it out. Probably she was just a good, discreet pharmacist.

See you next week, I said.

I hope not, she said. Or maybe I should hope so? Hope it helps.

I went home with my three pills.

What's that? asked my boyfriend.

Antidepressants.

How come? They think it's all in your head, right?

No, I said. These antidepressants affect how you perceive pain.

I don't get it, he said.

I was determined to try to explain it to him. Antidepressants work in the brain, I told him.

I know that, for Chrissake!

They affect the chemicals in the brain. The juices between the neurons.

My boyfriend just looked at me.

You know, I said, trying to sound authoritative. The brain works with electrical impulses and chemicals. If you change the chemicals, you change the functioning of the brain. That's what these drugs do.

They think it's all in your head, he said again.

In a way it is all in your head, I said. Your head is where you feel pain. I mean, your brain.

Why don't they give you some painkillers?

This is a kind of painkiller. It's a pain-perception killer.

I don't get it, he said. Why don't they give you some Percodan?

I don't want any Percodan.

You don't want to do anything about this, he said.

I went for a walk.

Why I Am Opposed
to Antidepressants

Because I think depression has something to tell me.

Because often depression is an appropriate reaction.

Because I am terrified of changing the functioning of my brain in any way.

Because I believe that depression is "me," and that without it I would not be "me."

Because I can't imagine my life without the time off I get from periodic depression.

These are the typical idiotic reasons people give for not wanting to feel better. So in this respect, I am quite normal.

The Brain, Part Two

My boyfriend was going to have dinner with his
parents in Rhode Island. I called Ingrid.

Can I come for dinner? I asked. I'm supposed
to take amitriptyline, and I don't want to do it alone.

How much? she asked.

Ten milligrams.

That's nothing! What's that going to do?

I don't know, Ingrid. Interrupt my pain circuitry.

We ate chicken paprika, and then I took a pill.

They do use it for chronic pain, Sanford said. Subclinical doses like that. Let's hope it does the trick.

We cleaned up and went into the living room.

I sat in my usual spot, the leather chair with the broken
front leg and the busted seat cushion that was draped in an
antique buffalo skin that Sanford had inherited from his
grandfather. I liked to run my fingers through the buffalo

fur. Masturbatory behavior, Ingrid had called it, once. I didn't care. It was like patting an inert dog—the perfect dog, that didn't drool or smell bad or complain if you stopped patting it. I also liked this chair because it was beside a good bookshelf, filled with titles like *Layard of Nineveh* and *Arabia Felix* and *Antique Kilims at the Metropolitan Museum.* On top of the bookcase were several Mexican papier-mâché figures of people with knives stuck through their heads and blood running down their faces, as well as an African wood statue of a man whose erect penis reached all the way up to his chin. I found these comforting, just like the buffalo skin, especially the people with the knives in their heads. They looked happy enough that way, and they were a nice metaphor for mental disturbance.

Sanford and I started to talk about what we were reading. I was reading about World War I. I'd just finished Siegfried Sassoon's *Memoirs of an Infantry Officer.* Sanford was reading about the lost city of Petra, in what is now Jordan, where he was planning to go in the fall. Ingrid took out the atlas so we could see where the lost city of Petra was.

How can it be lost if you're going there? I asked.

It was lost, said Sanford.

I can't find it, said Ingrid, picking up the magnifying glass.

As we were looking for Petra, I began to feel a peculiar sensation. At first, it was slight, a hint of something rather than something. I felt that most of me was sitting on the buffalo skin and looking at a map, but that some of me, the top of my head, let's say, was floating up near the ceiling, hovering above what was going on in the room.

I felt a brief spurt of alarm. Then the feeling passed.

We found Petra, and then we moved on to some reminiscences. Because Sanford and Ingrid have known me since I was two, they have all kinds of reminiscences of my childhood and my family, which, as I get older, I find more and more interesting.

But as we talked, a larger portion of my head became disconnected from the rest of me. I couldn't figure out exactly what this part of my head was doing. It was watching things from an odd angle. I didn't like it, and I got another surge of alarm.

I think I have a split consciousness, I announced.

Huh? said Ingrid.

Like some of me isn't *in* the conversation.

Hmm, said Sanford.

Well, said Ingrid.

It's okay, I said. I was trying to buck myself up. This is probably just the sensation of consciousness, I added. Then I wondered what I meant by that.

What do I mean by that? I asked them.

I don't know, said Ingrid.

We began talking about the man who used to be the principal of the elite and unpleasant high school I went to for one year, along with their son Paul, who'd managed to make it through four years. I hated this man, and he hated me, and I did not have a successful career in that school. He was an odd and obsessive person. Sanford and Ingrid were quite fond of him, though.

As I was recounting a particularly unpleasant incident with this man, who had accused me of going barefoot and become furious about it, when in fact I'd been wearing beige shoes, I began to have trouble remembering words. I couldn't remember the word *aggressive*.

He was very— I stopped. He was very assertive? I said. That's not what I mean, I said. Do I mean antagonistic? I thought about that. That was okay, but it wasn't the word I was looking for. I'm looking for a word, I said, but I can't find it.

Sanford nodded.

I started to panic. Hey, I said, I can't remember this word!

Happens all the time, said Ingrid.

But Ingrid, I said, you're eighty and I'm not. This word starts with a *p*, I said.

Paranoid? Sanford offered.

He was paranoid, but that wasn't the word, I said. My head was floating like a balloon. All of a sudden, I remembered the word.

Aggressive, I said. But it doesn't start with a *p*.

Sanford and Ingrid didn't seem to find this peculiar, but I did.

I'm going home, I told them. I'm nervous I won't remember how to drive.

I did remember how to drive, but I had to concentrate on it. When I got home I went to bed. It was around ten o'clock. I lay in bed and felt that I was being pressed down into the mattress. I felt heavy and flat and stupefied. This went on for hours.

Suddenly, my boyfriend was leaning over me. Hey, he was saying. You drunk? What's the matter with you?

Time. What's the time? I asked.

It's eleven, he said.

Oh God, I said. I couldn't seem to come out of the mattress enough to talk to him.

What's the matter with you, honey?

That pill, I said. I took. It.

Then I fell asleep.

In the morning I was still nailed to the bed. I had to keep instructing myself to get up. Eventually I did, but when I got downstairs I had to instruct myself about how to make coffee. Drinking the coffee didn't do anything for me. My head remained in a blur, while my stomach grumbled and tossed the coffee around.

One important fact: My vagina did not hurt.

In the afternoon, when I'd eaten a sandwich, things started to go back to normal. I washed the dishes and put the cheese in the refrigerator without considering every move. I also managed to read a few pages of a book. It was like coming out of a fever. I decided to call Ingrid.

I've been in a stupor ever since I left your house, I told her. Like novocaine in the brain. It's just wearing off. I was turned into a moron.

That's what my crazy patient says. Now I'm a moron! A *happy* moron. He's taking a hundred and twenty milligrams, though. And he's crazy.

I'm not crazy, I said. But I sure turned into a moron.

You're awfully drug-sensitive, said Ingrid.

I don't want to take any more of this stuff, I said.

I called the alternative nurse and explained what had happened.

I have to tell you, I said, that my vagina didn't hurt. But I couldn't function.

Don't take any more, she said. You can't be in that kind of state. Make an appointment for later in the week, and we'll see what we can do.

By that evening I felt like myself again, which made me all the more aware of how peculiar I'd felt on the drug. I wondered if I could be making it up. I decided not, because nobody had suggested to me that I would feel anything other than a dry mouth or some sleepiness. If the alternative nurse had told me I might feel my brain had been divided into a mostly nonfunctioning part and a small observatory segment, I would have been more suspicious of my reaction. Still, I was somewhat suspicious. I called Jamie.

Drug companies ought to test for side effects on you, he said.

Am I making this up? I asked.

How do I know? I'm not a doctor.

I always got irritated when he told me he wasn't a doctor. Technically, he was a doctor. Being a doctor is like being a Jew; you can't get away from it.

You are so a doctor, I said.

That conversation didn't go anywhere.

Two days later I was sitting in the alternative nurse's office again.

What about cortisone? I want to try cortisone.

It's not going to work, she said.

I want to try.

Okay, okay. You can try. She scribbled a prescription. It's not going to work. I want you to do biofeedback. That's going to work.

You said amitriptyline was going to work, I reminded her.

She laughed. For many people, it does. But let's try this. It's not a drug. It's not invasive. And I really think it's going to work.

I'm going to try cortisone first.

Here's the person to call, she said, handing me another

prescription sheet. She's at Saint Mary's. Report back to me after you've had two appointments.

After biofeedback doesn't work, what's left?

She didn't say anything for a few seconds. Then she said, Surgery.

I'm not having surgery.

Do the biofeedback, she said. It's going to work.

I put a big globule of cortisone cream inside my vagina when I got back from the alternative health center. Within an hour, my vagina felt worse, more irritated, and itchy as well. I was disappointed. Previous experience with the miracle of cortisone had made me expect to feel better. I called Saint Mary's. They were busy at biofeedback. The first appointment they could give me was in a month.

Over the next several days I polled my friends. Nobody had done biofeedback, not even Paula, who'd had back surgery. I associated back trouble with biofeedback—incorrectly, it seemed.

The doctor contingent was mostly for it.

Why not? said Laura next door. Might work. Won't hurt you.

Jamie was somewhat skeptical. If there's inflammation there's trouble, and I don't see why they aren't treating the inflammation.

Sanford and Ingrid had already weighed in on biofeedback as useful for pain.

My boyfriend wanted me to use the novocaine cream.

You won't even try, he said.

I did try, I said. It hurts.

Why won't you *do* anything about this!

My whole life revolves around doing something about this, I said. I go to some doctor or other almost every week.

Yeah, but nothing helps.

Well, that's not my fault, I said.

Why won't you have that surgery? That surgery works, right?

Why don't *you* have that surgery, I yelled. My vagina was yelling along with me, throbbing and stinging like crazy.

What's the point of going to a doctor and not doing what he says? He said he could fix it, didn't he?

Of course he said that. He's a surgeon. Anyhow, each doctor says something different. That's the problem.

He stormed out of the house.

I went over to see Paula.

She and Ettore were in the front room. He was standing at his table, painting and listening to Coltrane—this time, "Greensleeves." She was sitting on the sofa doing the accounts, with a heap of receipts and scrawled-on pieces of paper beside her.

What could this mean? she asked him. It was a scrap that said, Tuna fish and shellac.

Just what I had in mind for lunch, I said.

Shellac, said Ettore. I got some shellac. And the apprentice wanted a sandwich.

Do you have a receipt for it?

He pointed at the scrap.

From a store, said Paula. She sounded weary.

He shook his head.

She scrunched up the paper and dropped it on the floor, where there was a pile of scrunched-up paper.

What's the matter, honey? she said to me.

Everything, I said. I sat down next to the pile of receipts. We have the same conversation over and over. He wants me to have that surgery.

He's horny, said Paula. He wants you to be fixed.

Probably also he hates to see you miserable, said Ettore. It's scary when the woman is upset. He wants you to feel better.

But that surgery doesn't even work half the time, I said. Would you do that? I looked at Paula.

I bet I would. I had back surgery. That doesn't work either.

But it did work, I said. On you.

See? She grinned. That's not the point, she said. It's your decision.

I'm not doing it, I said.

Okay, said Ettore. That's settled. Forget about it. He'd

taken to saying Forget about it as if he were a wiseguy from Queens rather than a trompe l'oeil artist from Florence. He turned around from his table and said it again: Forget about it.

All right, Scarface, said Paula.

Coltrane was finished. Time for some ragas, said Ettore.

Oh no, not the ragas, said Paula. Let's go to the kitchen.

I like the ragas, I said.

They give me a headache, she said. Anyhow, I'm tired of these receipts—not that there are any.

Ettore pointed his paintbrush at the pile on the sofa. Receipts, he said.

You're right, she said. You're getting better.

We went to the kitchen.

Are you hungry? she asked.

No, I said. I'm too upset.

This relationship . . . said Paula.

I know, I said.

But really, don't you think some of it has to do with the relationship?

Yes, I said. And that gets me more worried. If I made it all up.

You didn't make it all up, said Paula. But maybe some of it. Or you indulge yourself in it. It gets you something.

I don't want to fuck anymore, I said. I can't. I don't even want to try. It's all too terrible. And that was the great thing for us.

I think your body is rejecting him, said Paula. You're sick of him, literally.

I'm certainly sick of him bugging me about sex.

He's not right for you, she said. He's worse than usual.

I didn't say anything.

Are you mad? she asked.

No, I said. You're not saying anything I haven't already said to myself.

I'm sorry it's all so bad, she said.

Oh, well, I said. Next stop, biofeedback. And after that? Saint-John's-wort? Crystals?

Why not? Laying on of hands. Buddhist chant.

Okay, okay, I said.

Gluten-free diet, she said. Pyramids—you can sit under a cardboard pyramid two hours a day. She was giggling.

I had to laugh too. Paula always ends up making me laugh.

We'll get those nuns who pray for people to pray for you.

What nuns? I asked.

Those nuns somewhere. They spend all their time praying for people, like with cancer. And the people with cancer get better. It's been documented. I mean with clinical trials.

Oh, come on, I said. I could imagine Jamie's look of disgust if I were to describe this experiment to him.

It's true, said Paula. The power of prayer.

They're not going to devote themselves to somebody with a sore vagina, I said.

I think you pay them. Contributions to their order.

Maybe I should just join their order, I said. I'm practically a nun already.

Biofeedback

In the middle of June, a year after I'd gone to my Italian gynecologist to complain about my vagina, I drove up the hill to Saint Mary's Hospital for my first biofeedback appointment.

The place felt familiar. When I got inside I knew why. It was a long-term-care hospital, and it had much in common with the psychiatric hospital where I'd spent two years of my youth. The drab green corridors scuffed at shoulder level from the pacers who dragged their bodies back and forth all day; the peeling plastic upholstery of the chairs where people sat whispering to themselves; the nurses with keys clanking at their waists, avoiding eye contact as they went on their rounds; above all, the pall of deep, still boredom that suffused every inch of the building, wrapping it in a cocoon of Nothing, Nowhere, and Never—all this made me feel at home.

The biofeedback area was painted the color of a paper bag. Booklets about urinary incontinence were piled on a plywood coffee table. There were also booklets from a drug company touting hormone-replacement therapy. Under one of these piles were a few Xeroxed flyers from the Vulvodynia Network: meetings in Somerville once a month; bring a casserole.

I waited about ten minutes. A young woman with a smooth triangular face and a bowl haircut popped her head out of a door.

I'll be right there, she said.

I waited another ten minutes.

She popped out again. Come in, she said.

The room was small and hot. A noisy box fan whirred on the floor beside a metal desk. A piece of medical equipment the size and shape of a toaster oven sat on a wheeled cart beside a narrow examining table. No window, no chair, not even a hook for my clothes.

I sat on the table and told my story. The biofeedbackologist nodded her tidy head.

Okay, she said. So what would you like to achieve from biofeedback?

Achieve? I asked. What do you mean?

Do you want to be able to resume intercourse?

No, I said. I was surprised to hear myself say this.

Do you want to be able to use other sexual techniques?

I didn't want to discuss sexual techniques with this person.

Listen, I said, I want to be able to drive a car without pain, to wear a pair of pants without pain, maybe even to use a Tampax without pain, and to sit around reading a book without pain. That's what I want.

This is very important to know, she said. If you wanted to be able to have intercourse, we couldn't say biofeedback had succeeded until you could do that. You see?

This was so self-evident as to be moronic. It was true, however, so I figured I'd go along with it. Okay, I said.

Put this on, she said, holding out a pale, limp hospital johnny, and I'll be back in a minute.

While she wasn't there, I considered the fact that I didn't want to be able to fuck. I didn't get very far in my consideration. The environment was not conducive to thought, I decided. I'd have to take the matter up under different circumstances.

When she came back in, she was rubbing her hands.

I would like to have permission to examine you, she said.

This also struck me as idiotic. Of course, I said. Isn't that why I'm here?

No. She shook her head. You're here for biofeedback. But I would like to examine you. Do I have your permission?

Yes, I said.

I need to ask you some questions first.

Okay, I said.

Have you ever had an abortion?

No, I said.

Have you ever had vaginal surgery?

Yes, I said. That Bartholin's cyst.

Have you ever been sexually assaulted?

No, I said. I wondered where she was heading.

Have you ever had sexual relations against your will?

Yes, I said, surprising myself again. I thought of my recent nights in bed with my tent and my boyfriend's insistent erection banging against my leg.

But still, you are giving me permission to examine you?

Get on with it, I thought, but all I said was, Yes.

If you're uncomfortable at any point we can stop.

I was already uncomfortable. Let's go, I said, lying back.

No. My examination is different, she said. I want you to sit up.

Her examination was indeed different. She seemed to be checking out my muscles. I hadn't known how many muscles there are in the vagina, so I found it interesting. A lot of them were sore.

Is this too intrusive? she asked.

It's peculiar, I said, but it's okay. Are you checking the muscles?

She nodded. She had one finger deep inside me. Her

other hand was on the outside, against my vulva, so she was pressing the vaginal wall between her hands. It didn't hurt much, but it was oddly intimate.

Squeeze, she said.

Eh?

Squeeze your muscles, like you're trying not to pee.

I squeezed.

Good, she said. That's quite good.

She took her hands away from me and stepped back. All right, she said. You have a lot of spasms. Spasm is a natural reaction to pain. Muscles protect themselves from pain by contracting. Unfortunately, spasm causes more pain. Which causes more spasm. I am going to train you to relax your vaginal muscles.

That sounds good, I said. But, I went on, the spasms are not the cause of the other pain, the tingling and burning, are they?

No, she said.

Then there's no way to fix that stuff?

This will help. The spasms maintain the tingling and burning.

But the tingling and burning came first, right?

She turned away and began to fiddle with the toaster oven. Then she rolled it over beside the examining table and pulled some wires out of the back.

Could you explain what you're doing?

This is the biofeedback machine, which measures the

strength of muscle contractions. It has skin sensors—she held up the wires—and they register on this graph—she pointed at a blur of lines on the screen of the machine.

I need my glasses, I said. I leaned over the examining table and got them out of my pocketbook, which was on the floor, because there were no hooks to hang my things on. Now I was ninety percent naked, wearing my glasses, and watching her glue wires to my abdomen.

Turn on your side, she told me. She stuck one of the wires into the crack between my buttocks. Now you can lie on your back again.

I was propped up on several pillows so I could see the screen of the biofeedback machine.

Now, squeeze, she said.

I squeezed.

Harder, she said.

I squeezed harder.

She pointed to the screen. See this bar? It goes up to ten. You want to squeeze it up to ten and hold it for ten seconds.

Where am I now? I asked.

You're at six.

I squeezed. Better?

That was eight, she said. And you're using your stomach muscles. Don't do that. Just use your vaginal muscles.

I had to concentrate on not using my stomach muscles.

It reminded me of being nine years old and trying to pat my head while rubbing my belly. Did I do it? I asked.

Yes, she said, but you're only at eight.

I focused all my energy on my next squeeze.

Good! she said. Hold that.

I can't anymore, I said. I let go.

All right, she said. But let go more. Relax more.

That was even more difficult. I pretended I was peeing, rather than that I was not peeing.

There you go, she said.

I was embarrassed to be pleased by her praise.

You want to go back to zero when you relax, she said. She pointed at the screen. Let's try it again. Get up to ten, like you did, hold it for ten seconds, then relax completely and hold it at zero for ten seconds.

It was like weight-lifting. I squeezed and held it for what felt like forever. Then I had to weight-lift in the opposite direction, somehow.

You're not looking at the screen, she said sternly.

I can't look at the screen while doing this, I told her.

All right. Do it again. I'll tell you when to start and stop.

More weight-lifting. Then: Relax! she said. When I felt that I had been relaxing for an hour, I started to squeeze again. Not yet, she said. Wait till I tell you.

We did this five times.

You have very good body awareness, she said.

Again, I felt inordinately pleased.

You can rent this machine, she said, but I think you'll be able to do it at home without the machine.

Good, I said. I didn't want to go home carrying a toaster oven that I would have to explain to my boyfriend.

Okay, she said. She peeled the wires off me, which hurt the way pulling off a Band-Aid hurts. Now, let's talk about the bladder.

The bladder?

She nodded her head. How many times a day do you pee?

I have no idea, I said.

Did you pee before this appointment?

I always pee before gynecological appointments, I said.

Did you pee before you left the house to come to this appointment?

Probably, I said. Or maybe I peed here. One or the other.

After this appointment, will you pee again?

I might, I said.

And when you get home, will you pee another time?

Not *both*. I wouldn't pee here and then pee again when I get home.

But you'll pee one of those times?

Probably, I said again. I guess.

Jicking, she said.

Huh?

Just in Case peeing. We call that jicking.

Who? Who calls that jicking?

She wouldn't tell me who called it that.

Do you always pee before you get into the car?

Listen, I said, if I have to pee, or think I will have to pee soon, I pee. I smiled at her. Didn't your mother always tell you to pee before getting in the car?

Your mother was wrong! She folded her arms across her chest. I am going to retrain your bladder.

I didn't want to have my bladder retrained. What's this got to do with what's wrong with my vagina? I asked.

It's all related. Do you pee at night?

You mean during the night?

Yes. Do you get up to pee?

Sometimes, I said. Not every night.

How many times?

Once. And it's usually early in the morning, like five-thirty.

Once *now*, she said ominously. It'll just get worse.

How do you know?

It always gets worse. She nodded. I am going to retrain your bladder, she repeated. When you pee, how long does it take to pee?

I was losing patience with this. I don't know, I said. What does it matter?

It matters, it matters. She nodded some more. When you pee, it should take eight Mississippis.

What are you talking about?

One Mississippi, two Mississippi, three Mississippi—eight of those. If it takes less than eight, you didn't have to pee.

How can *you* say *I* didn't have to pee?

Because I know, she said. She stood there with her tidy face and her crossed arms, staring me down. I know, she said again.

I don't think you can know if somebody else has to pee, I said, but I didn't feel sure of what I was saying.

She turned away and rummaged in one of the desk drawers. She pulled some things out and put them at the foot of the examining table. One was a small basin with prongs around it, and the other was a sheaf of papers.

This is an intake/outflow chart, she said, pointing at the papers, and this is a measuring container. Fits on the toilet. You note your intake on the left and the volume of production on the right.

Do I have to drink from a measuring cup? I asked. I was completely irritated.

No. You can measure the volume of one glass and use that glass only.

And what? I do this for a day?

No. You have to do this for a week. Bring it to your next appointment. It will show you how much you pee and when.

Then what?

Then I will retrain your bladder, she said, and left the room.

I got dressed, went into the hallway, found a bathroom, and peed.

When I got home, I peed again. I put the charts and the measuring device in my study, in the drawer where I kept the plastic dildo from the vulvologist and all the articles about my disease.

I didn't mention to my boyfriend that I'd been to biofeedback. I was too tired to have another one of our discussions. He was tired too, and he fell asleep before he could start to pester me to have sex with him.

My vagina was sore from all the prodding and weight-lifting. It was a tent night.

I dreamed I was having a big fight with my mother, and I woke up puzzled. My mother has been dead for a decade, and, for the most part, I've stopped dreaming about her. When I do, the dreams are friendly—which is not exactly how our relations were when she was alive. But of course, now that she's dead, I miss her.

The dream put me in a bad mood. I hid in my study and waited for my boyfriend to leave the house. I couldn't resist opening the drawer and looking at the pee charts. Seeing them made me angry.

I called Sanford and Ingrid.

Can I come for dinner? I asked.

Sure, come, said Ingrid.

Over the course of the day I peed at least a dozen times. I was doing it on purpose. I'd think about the biofeedback-ologist and her bowl of hair and I'd get angry, and then I'd pee. While I was peeing I'd feel I was getting revenge on her. I caught myself thinking things like, You can't tell me when to pee, and, How do you know when I should pee?, and, If I want to pee, I'm going to pee.

I also found myself counting the Mississippis. Early in the day I got up to five or six. But later, from all that unnec-cessary peeing, I was down to about two.

There was something sexual in the pleasure of peeing this way. I felt defiant and naughty and self-indulgent. But I felt lousy too: My bladder felt full when it wasn't, my vulva was stinging more than usual from wiping myself all the time, and the pain in my vestibule was radiating farther up into my vagina and also into the surrounding tissue, as if it had infected the entire peeing apparatus.

The worse I felt, the angrier I got. And I got worried, because I remembered a portion of the *Clinical Journal of Pain* article about cystitis and vestibular pain, which noted that bladder, urethra, and vagina all begin as the same cel-lular unit, the urogenital sinus, which during embryonic development differentiates, to some degree. But their cel-lular origins remain one, unlike other parts of the body—for instance, an ear does not have cellular kinship with an eye. This fact might account for my disease, they said, at least in some people, whose sympathetically maintained vaginal pain could be attributed to chronic bladder trouble. Probably, if I kept peeing at this rate, I would end up with chronic bladder trouble.

When I sat on the buffalo-skin chair before dinner at Sanford and Ingrid's that night, my crotch got too hot. I had to move to a wooden chair. I restrained myself and didn't talk about my vagina while they were having their vermouth. But as soon as we sat down to dinner, I launched into my latest installment.

As I described the biofeedbackologist and the anger she'd provoked in me, I realized what it was all about.

Hey, I said, I get it. She's trying to toilet train me. Or that's how I perceive it. That's why I'm so mad. I'm furious. As I said this I could feel my fury rising. I'm like a little kid who won't cooperate, I said. That's why I dreamed about my mother.

This realization amazed and delighted me.

It's as if I have a visceral memory of this, I went on. It's incredible. It's why I keep peeing. To assert my will against hers.

Isn't that something, said Ingrid.

Sanford also liked it. Hmm, he said, like a sense memory of toilet training.

I hate her, I said. I hate her. It was thrilling to say that I hated her. At the same time, I was aware of how silly it was to bother hating her, and how all of this really had to do with something else, from long ago.

Do you know what she is? I said. She's a Urinazi.

We got a good laugh out of that.

Maybe you can just ignore the peeing stuff and do the exercises, Sanford said. They might help.

But I'm afraid of her, I said. I'm afraid if I don't retrain my bladder according to her specifications she won't help me with the other things.

No! said Ingrid. She can't do that. She can't force you to do her ridiculous urinary things.

We'll see, I said.

To compensate for being uncooperative about pee, I did my exercises twice a day for the next four days. On the fifth day I noticed that my vagina was hurting more than usual. According to my pain diary from the previous month, at this point in my cycle things should have been fairly level, at about two plus. But I'd inched up above three. I decided to do the exercises only once a day. This worried me, though, because then I wouldn't have anything to offset the fact that I hadn't done my pee assignment.

Sitting on the biofeedbackologist's table again, I was tense, waiting for her to lecture me about peeing. I'd worked up a speech that made use of sentences like, I'm not comfortable with the bladder-retraining effort, and, I feel I need to focus on the pelvic-floor exercises—sentences I hoped would trigger the proper response in her New Age Urinazi mind. The proper response, of course, would be to "respect" my feelings.

She came in, pert, tidy, clean. Turn over, she said. Let's see how you did. She glued the wires to my ass.

Squeeze! she commanded.

I squeezed.

Excellent. That's very good. Now relax. That's not as good. Relax!

It's hard to relax when someone's yelling at you to relax. I tried to remember how my vagina would get loose and warm during sex, but that just made me sad.

You're not relaxing, she said.

Maybe I should start from a squeeze, I said.

We tried that. It worked a bit better.

It's all about control, she told me.

I tensed up immediately. I was sure she was going to start the pee lecture. But she didn't.

I drew a breath. Can these exercises make you feel worse?

Sometimes. She didn't look at me.

Is that because the muscles aren't used to it?

Could be.

But that will go away, right?

Mmm, she said. Do you do them every day?

Yes, I said. Now, I thought, she's definitely going to ask about pee.

Okay, she said. You're doing very well. See you in a week.

I felt kind of let down. I went into the bathroom down the hall for a quick pee.

I saw her on Wednesdays. By Saturday I was sure the exercises were making things worse. And I had another upsetting conversation with my boyfriend.

I was sitting on the sofa squeezing.

What are you doing? he asked.

Biofeedback exercises.

Let's see, he said.

You can't see. They're inside.

What do you mean?

Like trying not to pee. That's the exercise.

That's not an exercise, he said. Let me feel it.

No, I said. I tensed up.

Come on, he said. Just let me feel it. You never let me in there.

You've got me all mixed up, I said. I've lost track of my exercise.

I know a better exercise.

Better for *you*, I said.

We never fuck anymore, he said.

I can't!

You don't want to, he said. You don't want to do anything. If I had this disease, I'd still do everything I could to make you happy.

Maybe you wouldn't, I said. Maybe you wouldn't be in the mood.

I'm always in the mood, he said.

Unfortunately, this was true. It was one of the things I had loved most about him.

I decided to skip a day of exercise and see if I felt better. I didn't; I decided to skip another day. By Wednesday I'd skipped four days. I felt a little better.

Wednesday afternoon I was lying on the biofeedback-ologist's table.

Turn over, she said. She was holding her wires aloft.

Listen, I said, sitting up. I've got a problem with these exercises. They are making me feel worse. I stopped for four days and I felt somewhat better. It's as if the exercises irritate me more. Is that possible?

Yes, she admitted.

What can you do?

She didn't say anything.

What can people do if they can't do the exercises?

There are a few things, she said.

I waited.

What are they? I had to ask, since she wasn't telling.

Soaks, she said. She was mumbling.

Soaks? Like sitz baths?

Mmm.

Soaks of what?

Oatmeal, she said.

When I got home, I called the alternative nurse.

Alternative Health Again

Oatmeal, I said. I'm back to applying breakfast to my vagina.

The alternative nurse laughed. It helps that you keep your sense of humor, she said.

It doesn't really, I said. Well, maybe it does. Who knows. I sighed. This is the end, I said. There isn't anything more.

There's the diet.

I shook my head. I don't believe in that diet theory. The only thing on their Bad List that I eat regularly is lettuce, and I didn't get this disease from lettuce.

Right, she said. I'm not convinced about the oxylate theory either.

We were sitting in her office. For a minute or two, we sat in silence.

Maybe the psychological issues— she began.

But then I feel responsible! I started to cry. I feel it's hysterical. I feel that anyhow.

I know, she said. She came over to my chair and put her arm around my shoulder. Just cry, she said. It's all worth crying about.

I followed her advice. I cried for a couple of minutes.

Thanks, I said after I'd cried enough. I think I needed to cry *with* someone.

You could bring him in here, you know. Sometimes these guys need to have it explained to them.

I've explained it a million times.

But he might listen to me. I'm a professional, after all. She laughed.

I don't think he's going to listen to either of us, I said. He doesn't want to understand it.

He's got to, she said. He's got to learn to let you move at your own pace.

He can't, I said. Of course, this is why I fell in love with him—he's so emotional and sexual. Now look.

Yes, she said. Isn't it funny?

I felt at that moment that the alternative nurse and I were friends. Perhaps because of that, I said: I think he's forcing me to have sex with him.

You think? Don't you know?

I don't really know, I said. I guess I don't want to know.

Or I don't want to call it that. He pesters me every night until I give him a blow job or let him fuck me. I do it so he'll leave me alone. Is that forcing me?

It's a lot of pressure, she said.

He holds my head down, I said. He holds me down by the back of my neck. I could barely bring myself to tell her this.

That's not right, she said. And you know it isn't right.

Sometimes I feel that I'm choking, I said. But the blow job is better. When I let him fuck me, it hurts so much I can't bear it.

You know this isn't right, she repeated.

He says I should want to give him a blow job.

Do you?

No. Even if he didn't hold my head down I wouldn't want to. I want to forget about sex for months. I want to be left alone. I feel that if I were left alone, I could heal myself. If I didn't have to think about him and what he wants all the time. And he doesn't understand that it's all much more frustrating for me than it is for him. He can still have an orgasm—one way or another. I can't. I can't get *near* it. Whatever I do or he does, it hurts. It's hopeless. No wonder I want to forget about sex. I can't get any pleasure from it.

Bring him in here, she said.

I don't want to, I said.

Why don't you want to?

That's a good question, I said. I'll have to think about it.

Would you try Prozac? she asked me.

Absolutely not, I said. Anyhow, you told me it didn't work for this.

Amitriptyline works better, she said, but maybe for you Prozac would work. It's less stupefying. Also, things are so difficult, maybe it would help.

See, this is what I hate about Prozac, I said. My life is terrible, so I should take Prozac and feel better about it even though it's still terrible?

She grinned. But you could try it, she said.

Oh, all right, I said. Give me a prescription. I don't have to fill it. And if I fill it, I don't have to take it.

Just do what you feel you can do, she said. Call me whenever you want. Think about bringing him in here.

Prozac

ive me four, I told the pharmacist. I only want
four.

It takes at least two weeks to see an effect, she
said.

I'll see an effect in an hour, I said. I always do.

I took the bottle home and put it on my desk and
looked at it: Prozac, America's favorite drug. Here it was, in
my house. I picked up the bottle and shook it, listening to
the rattle of the pills against the plastic. Then I opened it
and looked at them. I thought of all the arguments I'd had
with my friends and my doctors and even with people I
barely knew about this drug. This drug was going to
change my life. This drug had changed their lives, or the
lives of people close to them, or the lives of their other
patients who were depressed. What was the matter with
me that I wouldn't try it? And so forth.

I sat there looking at the bottle. It was similar to standing at the edge of a pier looking down into deep, cold
water and debating whether to jump in. Or worse, like
standing on a cliff and debating whether to jump off. It was
also reminiscent of standing at Checkpoint Charlie—
something I'd done a few times back in the days of the two
Berlins—waiting to enter a country where I didn't want to
stay and wondering why I was going there. Part of what
made Checkpoint Charlie unnerving was the slight but real
fear that the "other side" might prevent me from crossing
back over, and that these were my last moments in the free
world.

My stomach hurt. And my chest hurt. The idea of taking Prozac made me so nervous that I was having trouble
breathing. I took out one pill and held it in my hand. I went
into the bathroom and got a glass of water and took it back
to my desk. Then I put the pill beside the glass of water and
looked at them.

I realized that I had to break up with my boyfriend. It
was the only way my vagina would have a chance to get
better. I didn't want to break up with him. I still loved him.
But he was driving me crazy and I couldn't make him stop it.

I put the Prozac back in its bottle. Then I put the bottle
in the drawer with my dildo and my pee basin. It had
worked. It had changed my life.

Internal Medicine Again

I'm not sick, I explained to Doctor Matthew's secretary on the phone. I just want to discuss something with him.

Can you wait two weeks? she asked. He's very busy.

That's fine, I said.

I made copies of all the articles about my disease and sent them to Doctor Matthew. I also sent a letter listing all the things I'd done about my vagina since I'd last seen him, in March. There were quite a lot: novocaine cream, amitriptyline, cortisone, biofeedback.

Every night my boyfriend pestered me to give him a blow job. Some nights I did. Even when I did, he pestered me to fuck too, or to give him another blow job.

It's not enough, he said. A blow job just isn't the same.

If it's not the same, how come you want two?

That made him mad. Because I need two, he said. You don't even like sex anymore.

You're right, I said. How could I possibly like sex anymore?

So, because you don't like sex, I'm not supposed to like it either?

Yes, I said. If you're having sex with *me,* and I don't want to, then I don't see why you want to.

I'm horny, he said. I want to have sex with you.

You're horny, I said, but I don't think you want to have sex with me in particular. You just want to have sex—any kind.

That's a big lie, he said. He looked really mad. This made me sure I was right.

Finally, it was time to go to Doctor Matthew.

I got your package, he said. That article from the *Clinical Journal of Pain* was very interesting.

Yes, I said. I thought that was the best.

So, what can I do? he asked me.

I'm not sure, I said. Did you get any ideas from reading that stuff?

I have a hunch, he said. It's just a hunch. My clinical instinct is it's a virus. Maybe nobody will ever isolate it, or prove that, but I think it's the most likely explanation.

So? I asked.

So, I could give you antiviral drugs.

Acyclovir?

Better. Not as unpleasant to take and a bit more effective.

What would it do?

It would reduce the viral load—if it's a virus. And then your symptoms might go away.

How long would I take it?

A couple of months. See if it got better. Then go down to some maintenance dose. It's worth a try.

I couldn't sleep when I took acyclovir.

This one might not have that effect.

But it might? I asked.

He raised his eyebrows. Only one way to find out, he said.

I didn't say anything.

Look, he went on, according to the criteria in these articles, you have this disease, syndrome, whatever it is. You fit all the conditions. It's real.

I still didn't say anything. I felt queasy.

Doctor Matthew— I started to say, but then I found I couldn't talk.

He sat there quietly.

Okay, this is what I want, I said.

Yes?

I want to stop trying to treat this, I said. I've been doing something about this for more than a year. I can't go on with that. I think I have to accept it as part of my life. If I could do that, I might relax, and then I might even get better. Somewhat better.

Relaxing would help, he said. It always helps.

I have to break off my relationship, I said. I hadn't said this aloud before. It's making everything worse. It's making me into nothing but this disease because my boyfriend is so focused on sex. I want to forget about sex and forget about my disease.

He stayed quiet, listening to me.

So, I went on, I don't know if I'll ever have another boyfriend. Who would love somebody who couldn't have sex?

It would have to be a particular sort of love, said Doctor Matthew.

I sat trying to imagine that particular sort of love. I couldn't.

Oh God, I said, I can't go on with this trying to fix it all the time. It might get better, right?

It could, said Doctor Matthew. Anything can happen.

I've become a vagina! I said. I can't stand it. There's got to be more to me than that.

He nodded.

So I don't want to take antiviral stuff, at least not now.

Okay, said Doctor Matthew. That's fine. If you ever want to, I'll give it to you.

Is it okay? I asked. Is it okay that I want to stop trying to fix it?

It's completely okay, he said.

I feel like I'm walking out on life, I said.

Part of it. For the moment, he said. But not all of it. As you said, there's more to you than a sick vagina.

I began to cry then. I'm so young, I said. I can't believe I have to say good-bye to sex already.

Doctor Matthew didn't say anything.

All right, I said, more to myself than to him. That's how it is. It isn't cancer. It isn't diabetes. It isn't life-threatening. It's just horrible.

There wasn't anything more for either of us to say.

Good-bye, I said to Doctor Matthew. I guess I won't see you soon. There's nothing else wrong with me.

You can call, he said.

We left it there.

Lust in Action

I had decided to break up with my boyfriend. I'd told Doctor Matthew I was going to break up with him. But I didn't do it. I didn't know how to do it. I wormed around it.

I saw my doctor, I said to him that evening.

What did he say? asked my boyfriend. He told you to have that operation, right?

No, he didn't. He told me he thought it was a virus.

Am I going to catch it?

This was an unforeseen response. I don't think so, I said, but I tried not to sound reassuring.

You sure?

Nobody knows if it *is* a virus, I said. My doctor thinks it might be.

So did he give you antibiotics?

Antibiotics don't kill viruses. They kill bacteria, I said. I was irritated with him for not knowing this. It's like the flu, I said. They can't fix the flu once you have it. It's a virus. Like AIDS.

You got AIDS? he asked.

No, no, I said.

I think you got AIDS. You fucked somebody else and you got AIDS.

That's ridiculous, I said. I didn't fuck anybody else. I don't have AIDS. This is some other virus—maybe.

Yeah? Well, where'd you get it? I don't have it. I didn't give it to you. Where'd you get it?

Nobody knows, I said.

Huh. He walked out of the room. Then he came back in. That was something he did when he was upset. Who'd you fuck? he asked me. Tell me who you fucked. You fuck Scott?

No, I said. You're not listening to me. I did not have sex with anybody.

You used to.

I used to have sex with you!

You fucked Scott.

During this conversation, my vagina was carrying on an internal monologue that went, Zing, sting, yow.

He went out of the room. When he came back in, he said, You're always over there with Scott, talking about books—you *say*. You're always over there.

We're talking about books, I said.

Huh, he said.

That night, a blow job for him and a tent arrangement for me.

I tried again the next evening.

My doctor and I have decided that the best thing for me is not to have any kind of sex for a while.

What's a while?

Months, I said. Months and months.

Nothing new about that, he mumbled. We haven't had sex for months and months.

What was that last night?

Goddamned blow job.

And that's not sex?

It's not my idea of sex. He scowled. If I had a sore dick, he said, I'd still fuck you. Nothing would make me stop fucking you.

But suppose it hurt so much you just couldn't do it?

It would have to hurt a lot. Like razor blades.

That's how much it hurts, I said. So suppose it hurt that much?

Then I'd eat you. Or whatever you wanted. I'd do *anything*. He moved closer to me. I'd do anything to keep you happy. Why won't you do that for me?

I have been, I said.

You have not. I have to tell you. You don't want to.

I didn't point out that these were three different objections.

It hurts, I said. I've explained that. Everything we do hurts.

You won't use that novocaine cream.

That stuff hurts worse, I said.

He turned around for a few seconds. Then he turned back and said, You don't love me anymore.

We don't seem to be making each other very happy, I said.

That is a dangerous sentence. It's penultimate—one more move and the world has changed. After I'd said it, everything stopped for a moment. It was a moment long enough for me to look both ways: back at all I'd hoped for from him and all the nights we'd spent in each other's arms, and forward to nothing I knew—to nothing, in fact.

You're ditching me, he said.

Are you happy? I asked. Nothing had changed yet.

Fucking ditching me.

I'm not happy, I said. And the air, which had been emptied out of me in that frozen moment, rushed back in. I can't stand this pressure anymore, I said. I can't!

Oh, he snarled, that's it. All I'm good for is sex. So now we can't have sex, you don't want me.

That's backward, I said. You can't leave sex alone.

Yes I can, he said. I haven't fucked you for months.

More like a week, I said. But the argument was over.

In bed that night a pernicious nostalgia came over us both, as it often will at these times.

You'll have to find another place to live, I said. But you can stay until you do.

Oh, honey, I don't want to leave you, he said He began to cry. I don't want to. Can't we try again?

He began to kiss me. The pain of parting was so great that it overcame the pain in my vagina, and we kissed each other as we hadn't in nearly a year. Everything about him fit me and felt right: how my legs could wrap around him easily because he was so slim and straight, how our arms slid down each other's backs and flanks, how his warm, taut weight rested on my hips and shoulders, a familiar burden whose very pressure stirred me.

Just a sec, he said suddenly, and hopped out of bed.

It had been a long time since I'd lain in bed longing for him. The thrill of that—the abandonment to a pleasure to come—was something I'd forgotten, though we had often indulged in it, interrupting ourselves to go downstairs and smoke a cigarette, for instance, to savor the postponement, the anticipation, the desire so sharp that sometimes I would press myself against a chair to urge it on or quell it or both at once, while he smoked and watched me, grinning.

In bed that night, waiting for him to return to me, I let my awareness drift, briefly, to my vagina and its sensations, checking—but doing it under my breath, so to speak—to see if it hurt. I was afraid if I focused on it, it would hurt. But it didn't. It was as if arousal had cured it, as if the pleasure had short-circuited the pain, the way rubbing your foot when you stub your toe makes your toe hurt less. The brain can feel only one sensation at a time. But I didn't want to think about it, so I stretched my arms out against the sheets and thought about my boyfriend's hips and how tightly I would grip them.

He came back and stood beside the bed. His right arm was at a peculiar angle to his body, and he was holding his hand aloft. Instead of lying down beside me, he sat on the edge of the bed near my knees.

What are you doing? I asked him.

He didn't answer, and I felt a flash of worry.

I looked at his hand, which was pointing at me, and I saw that the index and middle fingers were shiny, coated in something viscous that was dribbling down toward his palm.

What's that? I asked.

It's that novocaine, he said.

No, I said. I don't want that stuff. That stuff hurts a lot.

I want to fuck you, goddamnit, he said, lunging at me, pushing his hand between my legs.

I jumped out of bed. I was naked, and though it was a summer night, the air felt chilly. There was a streak of novocaine cream on my inner thigh. I ran downstairs. All I could think of was to get away from the bed and from him and his fingers. I pressed my back against the wall of the living room and shook, from cold and the remnants of my desire, and wondered if I should go next door to Scott and Laura because, I realized, I thought he might rape me.

For a short time I indulged myself in this idea. He was trying to rape me. But he wasn't really, was he? I'd been more than willing five minutes earlier. That was the point, though. That was why I felt he was trying to rape me. Because he hadn't seen how willing I was. All he could see was what he wanted.

I heard him moving around above me. I could put on my raincoat, I thought, and just run next door. Even considering this frightened me. I couldn't tell if it was self-preservation or hysteria. I decided I would leave if I heard him coming down the stairs. I didn't. I stood poised against the wall for quite a while, listening.

Then I got too cold and too tired to keep standing there. In the hall closet was a blanket, and I tiptoed over to get it. Then I tiptoed to the sofa and curled up under the blanket, shivering. The tiptoeing had made me nervous again. It confused me, just as debating whether to go next door had confused me. Was I in some sort of danger or not? Probably not, I thought. Then I imagined that he'd come downstairs and was leaning over me, and I felt a zing of fear. Eventually, though, I fell asleep.

I woke up at dawn. I could hear the shower running. Taking a chance, I dashed upstairs and grabbed my clothes from the day before. I couldn't face whatever was coming without clothes. I scrambled into them in the living room—just in time, because then he came downstairs.

I woke up and you weren't there, he said.

I slept here, I said. My voice was hoarse.

Honey, he said. He moved toward me.

I moved back. No, I said. Listen, I'm going away for a few days and I want you to leave.

What do you mean? Where are you going? You said I could stay.

I don't think so anymore, I said. I could tell I was wavering, though. To keep myself in line, I thought of his fingers coming at me. I've changed my mind, I went on, and I want you to go now. Tonight, or tomorrow at the latest.

Where are you going? he asked again.

Never mind, I said. I had no idea where I was going.

Did I do something? he asked me.

I stared at him. He didn't know; I could see that. He didn't think he'd done anything unusual or bad. This fascinated me. I was riveted by the fact that we could see things so differently. Then, like a seepage, the possibility that he hadn't done anything unusual or bad rose up in my mind. At the same time, everything he'd ever done had a new quality to it now, since it had been done by someone who could—or maybe even did—try to rape me.

If that was what he'd been doing.

You'd better go to work, I said. I turned my back on him, conscious that I was doing it, and went upstairs to take a shower.

No Consensus

Did you want to have sex with him? Laura asked.
I'd gone next door. Luckily, Laura was taking a
day off from her practice.

Yes, I said, but not with novocaine.

Did you say that?

Yes. I told him I didn't want to use it because it made
things hurt more.

And did he go ahead anyhow?

He tried, I said.

Did he manhandle you?

Manhandle, I said, that's an interesting word.

Forget about that stuff, she said sharply. Did he?

He wanted to jam it in me, I said.

Jamming, not listening—what does that sound like?
Doesn't that sound like forcing someone?

Hearing her say it made me doubt it.

Don't let him back in the house, she said. Things could get worse. I've seen some terrible things, you know.

I didn't doubt that.

Why don't you stay here for a couple of days, she said.

I was hoping I could, I said.

Laura took hold of my hand, which was very doctorly of her, and said, You stay here, and we can all keep an eye on him, see when he moves out.

She went to the gym and I went to see Paula.

Boy, is he bad, Paula said. Bad. Well, you always liked that about him. A bad boy.

Was he raping me? I asked her.

Impolite, she said. That's no way to treat a lady.

I told him to move out, I said.

Good, said Paula. You knew he wasn't the right one, didn't you?

I don't know anything, apparently, I said. I've got the creeps.

About him?

About myself, too.

She opened the refrigerator. We could have some scaloppine left over from last night. Oh, here's some chicken and rice soup I made yesterday before I decided to make scaloppine instead. Want that?

What's for dessert? I asked. Paula's specialty is dessert.

I made a wonderful melon sherbet, but we finished it. I've got a tea cake. It's from the store. It's old.

How old?

Monday. She picked it up and squeezed it. It's fine. Let's toast it.

We had soup, with toasted tea cake, which was a good combination.

How many years have I been sitting in your kitchen eating lunch and crying over some boyfriend? I asked.

At least twenty by now.

I'm never going to grow up, I said.

What do you want to do? Buy a four-wheel-drive vehicle and move to Concord?

No, I said. I mean something else. Even you got married.

Gee, thanks, said Paula. You don't want to get married, she said.

Are you sure?

If you wanted to get married, you wouldn't have picked him. Or any of the other ones.

Do you believe that personal responsibility stuff? You don't, do you? It's crap, I said. You can't argue with sexual attraction. It's like having to pee.

Fine, go to bed with him, she said. That's not the problem. Why did you let him move in with you, for God's sake?

I was lonely. I loved him.

Did you really love him? she asked me.

I have no idea, I answered.

That evening I called Maria from Scott and Laura's house.

But he didn't hit you? she asked.

No.

Thank God for that. You'd better stay at Scott and Laura's.

I am, I said. That's why I called, to tell you where I am. He never hit me, I went on. He wouldn't do that.

You don't know. People are capable of anything.

Oh, come on, I said. But Maria knows a thing or two—not just about molecular biology. She grew up under the Communists in Poland, that tragic country chewed at by its neighbors for centuries. Then the war, then the second war and her father in the camps. She got some data un-available in Cambridge.

Don't worry, I said. I'm safe here. I'll talk to you to-morrow.

Scott made potato pancakes for dinner. He made apple-sauce too. After the kids had gone to bed, he said, You ought to bring charges against him.

For what? I said. Being an asshole?

From their kitchen windows, through the curtains—plain, as I'd suggested—I could see the lights shining in my house. It looked inviting over there, and I felt ridiculous for having exiled myself.

Maybe I should just go home, I said. Maybe I'm making too much of this.

That would be a big mistake, said Laura.

You're nuts, said Scott.

I had a hard time getting to sleep that night. My vagina was burning and throbbing from all the upset. And I was unused to sleeping alone. I missed my boyfriend. I lectured myself about missing him: If he were here, I told myself, he'd be poking his dick into your back or your thigh, trying to fuck you. Then he'd be whining and pleading, or, who knows, forcing himself on you. But this lecture made me feel worse, because it made me despise myself for missing him, and for loving him in the first place.

The worst part, though, was the question of whether he'd tried to rape me. What was so terrible about his wanting to stuff novocaine cream into my vagina? How was that different from stuffing his penis into my mouth when I didn't want it there? It wasn't different.

The difference was, I'd resisted. And that showed me what he was doing. He'd been doing it for nearly a year, but I'd gone along with it. I knew what was happening.

I thought of the biofeedbackologist asking me if I'd ever had sex against my will, and of answering yes, and of telling the alternative nurse that he was coercing me into giving him blow jobs, and I wondered what exactly I had been thinking when I said those things. I supposed, lying in Scott and Laura's guest room in the attic, that I hadn't been thinking. I had just been feeling. But I couldn't even remember what I'd been feeling.

Maria seemed to be correct in her assertion that people are capable of anything.

Alone

Saturday night there were no lights on in my house. On Sunday Scott went over with me to see if my boyfriend had taken his things. He had. His tool chest that had sat behind the house, with his miter box and his router and his planes and his handsaws inside, his pile of odds and ends of lumber tucked into a blue tarp, his six-foot ladder made of nonconducting fiberglass—all gone. The closet in the bedroom was lopsided, my clothes listing to the left, making room for his clothes, which weren't there.

I was free to go home, where I could be alone with my sore vagina.

It'll get better now, said Paula. It was a psychological thing.

Maria agreed. So did Scott. Laura wasn't sure. Ingrid and Sanford also temporized. I noted that the doctors' prognoses were less rosy. Jamie declined to give an opinion.

My vagina remained sore. It was somewhat improved, because it wasn't irritated by unwanted attentions. On a scale of zero to five, it stayed around two. If I had to drive a lot, or if I got overtired, it would edge up past three. But then it would subside, to two. It didn't go below two.

My friends assumed I was cured. My boyfriend was gone, and since he had been the source of the problem, the problem was solved. When I complained that my vagina hurt, they thought I meant it hurt a little right then, that evening. They didn't seem to understand that it hurt all the time.

As long as I'd been living with my boyfriend, I could hope things would improve when I was living alone. Now I was living alone, but there was no improvement, and I had more time to think about how my vagina hurt. The fights and reconciliations and the pestering and the need to explain everything over and over had distracted me from the pain even though all those things had made the pain worse.

Low-grade pain is debilitating in a subtle way. I could get interested enough in a movie or a conversation to forget about the pain for an hour or so, but it lurked just beyond consciousness. I tried tricking it. Go away! I'd tell it, or, I'm not paying attention to you. I could feel my body tensed, though, waiting for the return of the pain. And of course, it always returned.

The fact of the pain was the burden. This fact was like an unwieldy piece of luggage that I had to drag around.

When I went out to dinner, or took a walk, or got into bed, I had to slog the luggage along with me. The pain itself was not that bad. What was bad was the idea that I was stuck with it. There was no checking it, or storing it in the over-head bin, no unpacking it and putting it in the closet, and that was what sapped my energy.

The Dead Vagina

This went on for months and months, though some days the pain was much less. Then, in the early spring, there came a week in which my vagina did not hurt. It had somehow regained the capacity to be normal—that is, to feel nothing. It still got agitated and zinged and stung, but it had remembered how to calm down to zero.

I wondered if it had remembered how to feel good, too.

I poked around at it. It was like poking at my foot—actually, it was like poking at somebody else's foot. There was no sensation at all. My vagina had curled up into itself like a hedgehog, cool, dry, and unresponsive.

I didn't know what to do. Rent X-rated movies? Buy a dildo? I had a dildo, I remembered, a gift from the vulvologist. It was clear plastic and resembled a turkey baster. It probably *was* that thing referred to as a turkey baster used in artificial insemination routines. It did not appeal to me.

Nothing did. My vagina had died.

I shouldn't have been surprised. I'd killed it. First I'd banished it to the edge of my awareness, where its endless complaints wouldn't bother me too much. Then I'd forbidden it to express interest in any person or activity, because I knew if I indulged it, it would start up with that zing, sting stuff again. Exiled, starved, and in solitary confinement, it had eventually succumbed.

I noticed some other things had died as well. When I went to the movies and saw enormous beautiful people kissing each other or getting into bed with each other, I drifted into a zombielike state in which the images didn't register on my eyes. The same thing happened when I came to romantic passages in novels. I simply didn't take them in. I was like one of those new TVs programmed to block sexy scenes. I didn't even want to hear about the ups and downs of my friends' marriages and love affairs. The entire continent of human attachment had become Australia: far away and incomprehensible.

That's not true, said Maria when I complained to her about this. You're attached to your friends. We love you.

It's different, I said.

Well, it's not *sex*. She laughed. But you can't say it isn't attachment. Probably, it's the only attachment you can count on. She was having boyfriend trouble.

Sex really is the basis of everything, I said. It's not that you have to act on it, but when eros goes away, life gets dull. It's as if I'm colorblind. The world is gray.

Somebody will come along and it will change, said Maria.

How can anything change? I wailed. How can anything change at all? I have a dead vagina. It can't feel anything except pain. And people can tell.

Don't be ridiculous, said Maria.

But people could tell. Nobody ever caught my glance on the street, or came up to me at a party, or tried to engage me in conversation in a bookstore. I was emitting something that kept people away. Or maybe I was not emitting whatever draws people together. The technicalities didn't matter; I was turning into ectoplasm.

Every couple months I'd investigate my vagina. It was usually still dead. Sometimes it would say hello to me, opening up and secreting a few drops of something that resembled tears more than the slick of arousal. Once or twice when it did that, I insisted on wringing some further response from it. The results were not very gratifying, and the aftereffects—the cheese grater, the stinging, the tent arrangement—lasted almost two weeks.

Nearly a year had passed since I'd told Doctor Matthew I wanted to forget about sex. I have to say good-bye to sex, I'd said. And although when I'd said that, it made me sad, I'd had no idea what it would be like in actuality.

In actuality, I couldn't say good-bye. All I'd done was remove myself from the arena of sexual behavior. Sex was everywhere, making fools of everyone and churning up the order people tried to bring to their lives, while I watched from my peaceful, tidy, inert, dead sideline.

I envy you, said Maria. Look at all the misery you're avoiding. What a waste of time, worrying over a man.

But I knew she didn't mean it. What she meant was she wanted to get along better with her boyfriend. She wanted to feel safe in his love and desire for her, or to find another boyfriend who could make her feel safe.

Infantilized, I said to Ingrid. That's what I feel. Not even—an infant is sexier than I am.

Latency, she said. Eight or so.

That's such a nice time of life, said Sanford.

It's only nice if you're eight! I protested.

Sometimes I felt that I was eight, though. In my quiet, clean house, where no man came bumbling in with demands or dirt or noise, where the table next to the sofa was stacked with books I wanted to read and the refrigerator was supplied with food I liked to eat and the sheets on the bed were fresh, I had a sense of contentment and control that reminded me of childhood. I remembered winter afternoons organizing my collection of glass animals and making cutout snowflakes with an eight-year-old conviction that I ran the entire world and could arrange it to my liking.

In the decades since then I'd learned that I didn't run the world. Like everybody, I'd learned all sorts of dreary things about the world and myself in it. The worst, of course, was the fact that I was going to die. It was actually going to happen to me. Not that I quite believed it—but the older I got, the more I saw that everything I did was just a protest against death, a heaping up of weight on the life side of the balance so that maybe, somehow, death wouldn't be heavy enough to take me.

But death had gotten a grip on my vagina. What an irony, when sexual delight is one of the main compensations for mortality. He wasn't much of a lover, death. He was the lousiest lover I ever had, but he clung to me like nobody else. In his cold, immobile attentions, he outdid even my boyfriend.

I wanted my vagina back.

I wanted unpredictability, upset, waywardness. I wanted the world to regain the other dimension that only the vagina can perceive. Because the vagina is the organ that looks to the future. The vagina is potential. It's not emptiness, it's possibility, and possibility was exactly what was missing from my life.

Homeopathy

And then I met a man who pleased me.

He was much taller and younger than I, and he came with a lot of accessories, such as earrings and tattoos and a motorcycle. He was clean and healthy, and he had been carefully raised in a good family and educated in fine universities, and no tattoos could obscure all that.

He appeared at my house, announced by the rumble of his motorcycle, on summer evenings when the light was long, and we sat on the porch and talked about books and the friends we had in common and what we were writing or having trouble writing. Then he'd rumble off again to romantic—or perhaps merely erotic—encounters scheduled for later.

My vagina liked him too.

At first it was just a wisp of a feeling, a tightening and lifting inside that occurred when he put his hand on my shoulder or said something I particularly enjoyed. As we approached midsummer, the feeling began to consolidate, so that being with him took place on two levels—the external in which we sat on the porch and talked, and the internal in which my vagina thrummed along making conversational overtures to his long legs and his fine clean hands.

I didn't know if his legs and hands were talking back to my vagina. Sometimes I thought they were. He often looked at me in ways that my vagina recognized. He was likely to disappear for a while after that happened. Then I'd sit on the porch alone and ponder the mysteries of desire.

My life was different with a revived vagina. It was upset, unpredictable, and wayward, just as I'd wanted it to be. At times I missed the peace of the dead vagina. But there was a lot of energy in desire. It simmered in me, frizzling and trembling in a way that reminded me of how my vagina had simmered in pain when it was ill. This proximity of pleasure and pain was confounding.

Desire—mine for my boyfriend, and his toxic, incessant desire for me—had made me ill. Maybe, desire would be my cure.

I cultivated my yearning, out of necessity. I had only my yearning to heal me. I used it to reclaim my vagina. It was difficult. My vagina was scared and shy, and my approaches to it were tentative. Often, when I first touched it, I felt the zing of pain. I began to realize that something

SUSANNA KAYSEN

had gone wrong with my perceptions. I'd learned, from two years of discomfort, to register any sensation as pain. Now I had to learn to suspend this perception of pain and press on through it to pleasure.

And pleasure was there, waiting for me. I'd been unable to find it before because my desire had been disembodied and theoretical. It wasn't disembodied anymore. There was more than six feet of it, stretched out on my sofa or leaning against my refrigerator while I made dinner, blue-eyed, soft-voiced, and lovely with the luster of my yearning for him.

I didn't dare say anything to him. Partly, I wasn't sure of my vagina. Perhaps it would yelp in pain if anyone else touched it. Partly, I wasn't sure of him. I wasn't even close to sure.

I called Paula.

It couldn't be, I said, that I want him this much and he doesn't want me. Right? That wouldn't be possible.

Are you crazy? she said. What do you think most novels are about? Wanting somebody who doesn't want you back.

She was right, as usual. I'd even written a novel like that.

But he keeps coming around here, I said.

He likes you. You're good company.

Good company! That's humiliating.

Hey, she said. You're a million years older than he is.

Only half a million, I said. He's a grown-up.

· 130 ·

A grown-up with earrings.

You sound like our parents complaining about bellbot-toms and long hair, I told her. Earrings are nothing. They all wear earrings these days.

Fine, she said. I could tell she was irritated. Then she said, Maybe you're practicing for the real thing.

Now I was irritated. There is no goddamned real thing, I said. You and your real thing. This is as real as it gets. He walks in the door and I get wet.

That's nice, honey, she said. Just enjoy that.

It was the day after midsummer, the top of the arc of the year. We were going to a movie on the other side of town.

I got onto the motorcycle behind him. Usually, I held on to his belt loops, but that night he was wearing pants that had none. I slid my thumbs inside his waistband and gripped it in my fists. His skin was warm against my wrists, and I could feel the edges of his hipbones shifting as he moved his weight with the motion of the bike.

I think I'll take Memorial Drive, he said, when we stopped at a light. It's faster.

It's a beautiful road that runs along the river, curving with it past the city spread out on the opposite shore. The light was failing slowly, washed out from the heat of the day. He speeded up. The wind whipped me so hard my eyes started running. He kept going faster, and I got scared. I thought how dangerous it was, what we were doing, and I tensed my legs a little around him.

Relax! he yelled, turning his cheek back toward me. I know what I'm doing.

My vagina did a somersault. He'd felt me tensing, through the fabric of his clothes and mine and through the noise and shaking of the motorcycle. Probably he could sense what was going on in the middle of me too. I felt caught out. But I felt triumphant as well. Now I knew that our bodies talked to each other.

Then he made a left off the river road and dipped so deep into the curve that I tensed again.

Don't fight me on the curves! he yelled.

Right then I thought, He will be my lover. It was the intimacy of that instruction—the sort of thing a lover says in bed, pressing his face into your neck, Don't fight me, darling—that made me sure.

We were coming to another turn. I let myself open up to him. I relaxed my legs—after all, he was there, where I wanted him, right between them—and loosened my grip on his waistband and let gravity and his body's hold over mine keep me steady through the curve. We shot through it together, everything inside me tumbling and the night air streaming around us like a huge dark kiss.

I leaned forward and put my chin on his shoulder. Better? I asked him.

Much better, he said.

How This Story Should End

This is what I want, I say to him. I want you to come to me completely naked. Take out your earrings, take off that silver ring on your index finger, take the watch and the bracelet off your arm, undo that string around your neck, take off your clothes, and come to me with nothing at all between us. That's how I want you, I say to him. Absolutely naked is how I want you.

We're in the kitchen. He looks at me and doesn't say anything. Then he takes the ring off. It clatters onto the counter. The watch and the bracelet, and the leather string from around his neck follow the ring with a clink and a soft thud. He starts to fiddle with the earrings. I never take these out, he says. You're taking them out now, I tell him. I have the impulse to help him—it's difficult to remove earrings without a mirror—but I don't want to touch him yet.

I have a navel ring, he says. Shall I take that out too?

Let me see it, I say.

He pulls his T-shirt up an inch. It's a tiny hoop. His navel is also tiny, a flat half-moon on his belly.

Take it out, I say. All these decorations, you don't need them.

I like them, he says. He puts the navel ring on the counter, on top of the pile he's made there. Then he says, You like them too.

He's right about that. The idea that he knows I like them makes me shiver with pleasure, because it means he knows things about me that I don't tell him, which could include all sorts of things we're going to do.

Okay, he says. He points at me. You too.

I take my earrings out. I take my two rings off. I add them to the pile. My things are gold; his are silver. It's quite a trove of jewelry we've got there.

Without my rings, my hands feel new and exposed.

I feel stripped, I say. I feel—

I'm in his arms. I don't know how this happened. I don't remember moving there. He smells clean, and his body is so warm that I flush from being near it. I've forgotten the warmth that comes off another human being. His blood is beating in his neck under my cheek, slamming against his veins. I put my hands around his rib cage and the force of life, the heat and noise of it, assaults me. We don't kiss. I am too overwhelmed to kiss him. I will faint if I kiss him. I wonder if he feels the same.

He pushes me away a little.

He's sitting on the kitchen stool and I'm standing in front of him. In these positions, we are almost the same height. He looks younger without all his geegaws.

What was the rest of the plan? he asks. Take off my clothes?

Eventually, I say. My voice is weak.

His knee is propped on the rung of the stool, level with my hips. He knocks it into my thigh several times, gently, reeling me in toward him until I'm standing between his legs. He puts one of his hands, the one that no longer has a ring on it, under my shirt onto my back and presses his palm against my spine.

I can barely keep standing up. On the other hand, I don't really need to stand up, because I am floating or pivoting around my vagina, which has become the fulcrum of my existence. I am suspended on it, on the heat and wetness of it, and I no longer feel my legs or my feet or the kitchen floor.

Aren't you going to kiss me? he says.

My mouth is so dry I can't imagine kissing him with it. There's another reason I hesitate. The moment before you kiss someone is the best moment of all, and I want to extend it. Once you've kissed, once you've tasted each other, entered each other's bodies, the entire business has been concluded in some way. This is why a kiss equals an infidelity. A fuck is just a full-body kiss. The kiss is what breaches the separation between two people. Nothing is ever the same after a kiss.

I run my tongue over my lips, but everything is like sandpaper. I don't understand how I can be so dry above and so wet below. I feel that I cannot breathe and that in fact I am not breathing. He's only two inches away from me. I can't seem to close the gap between us, though.

I manage to put my mouth against his mouth. He opens his mouth and breathes into me, and then he starts talking to me, with his lips moving against me.

Are you afraid? he asks. I'm afraid, I guess, he goes on, but while he's talking, he's licking my lips and biting them a little, and my mouth is no longer like sandpaper at all but as soft and wet as the rest of me.

Why are you afraid? I ask him.

Now everything will change, he says, and we stop talking and everything changes.

An Error

B ut my vagina and I were wrong. That young man did not desire me.

He was pretty blunt about it, too.

I thought you liked me, I said.

Oh, I really like you, he said. But I don't like you that way.

We were in the kitchen. He was sitting on the stool. He was wearing his ring and his bracelet and his watch and his earrings and the string around his neck. It was August, and the summer was fading. I could feel it running out.

Are you hurt? Do you not want to be friends?

I'm stung, I said. I didn't want to say more. We can be friends, I said. After all, we are friends.

Of course, I was hurt. For a while I was preoccupied with that. I lay on my sofa and felt rejected. I'd spent plenty of time that way in my life, so it was familiar. Something about it, though, was unfamiliar and scary.

It took me a week or so to figure it out.

My vagina had not made this sort of mistake before.

I had. I had thought one man still loved me when he didn't, and I had thought another man loved me more than he did, and I had thought a third man would leave his wife for me, and I had thought all sorts of incorrect things women think about men. But my vagina had never been wrong.

When my vagina said, He wants me, he—whoever he was—wanted me, whether he did anything about it or not. And whoever he was and whatever he did, he would always admit to wanting me.

Now I couldn't rely on any of my vagina's perceptions. This was even worse than its inability to distinguish pleasure from pain. That problem might be fixable, but I wasn't going to find anyone to fix it with me if my vagina had gone blind as well and couldn't tell who was a promising candidate.

A Fundamental Inequality

Paula and I were making stuffed cabbage for the new year. We had a bowl of spiced meat, two boiled heads of cabbage cooling on the breadboard, sweet-and-sour tomato sauce on the stove, and a large casserole waiting to be filled. We did this every September. We always ran into the same problems.

The cabbage leaves that were big enough to fill and roll successfully were too hot to handle. Farther into the cabbage the leaves were cooler but less cooked, which meant they were stiff and hard to deal with. At the center, the leaves were so small we could barely get any meat into them.

Look at this eeny-weeny one, I said, holding it up. It fell apart. Maybe that's too small, I said.

Jam it in on the side, said Paula.

The second head wasn't cooked enough. I peeled off

each leaf and handed it to Paula, who dropped it in boiling water for another five minutes. Eventually we had three plates heaped with poached cabbage. Then we had to wait for the leaves to cool.

Let's have a cigarette, said Paula.

We sat at the table smoking, the smoke rising up along with the steam from the cooling cabbage.

Still depressed over that boy? she asked.

My vagina's lost its mind, that's what depresses me, I said. How could it have been so completely wrong?

People make those mistakes all the time.

Not me, I said. I've never made this mistake before.

At least it's working, she said. It got all juiced up for him.

What good does that do if he doesn't want me? Anyhow, now it hurts again.

It's insulted, said Paula. But honey, you shouldn't be surprised. The young want to be with the young.

You think it's just the age thing?

Paula laughed. Look at us!

We're not that bad, I objected.

I was wearing a shapeless T-shirt with a big olive-oil stain down the front. Paula was wearing a brown vest of Ettore's that he didn't like because it didn't look good on him; it didn't look good on her either. Each of us had lost a molar to a failed root canal earlier in the year. I had arthritis of the right thumb and index finger. In the mornings they looked like little stuffed cabbage leaves, puffy and tight. Paula had developed a tendency to break her left ankle: three fractures in the past eight years.

But when I looked at her, I saw the sixteen-year-old girl I'd met in tenth grade, with her aureole of fair hair and her dazzle of freckles and her beautiful milk-white arms.

We're pretty bad, said Paula. I wouldn't want to fuck us.

Ettore wants you.

We're married, she said, as if that explained everything. You know, she went on, sex gets less important.

Maybe for you, I said. And that's because you have him. If there were no Ettore, wouldn't you spruce yourself up and go out looking for someone?

I might not bother, she said. And look who's talking.

We're making stuffed cabbage, I said. I'm supposed to put on high heels for that?

You haven't gotten dressed up in years.

Oh, I see, I said. If I wore lipstick, that kid would want me? Is that the idea?

Might help.

I never wore lipstick, and I never had trouble finding a boyfriend.

Paula picked up a cabbage leaf and put a few spoonfuls of meat in it. They've cooled down, she said.

You think I should cool down too, right?

She didn't say anything.

You think it's unseemly that I want that young man, don't you?

It's unlikely, she said. More than unlikely—he told you he doesn't want you.

I slapped the table with a wooden spoon. Men do it all the time, I said. Think of all the men cavorting around with women twenty years younger.

They're men. She handed me a cabbage leaf.

There is something icky about it, isn't there? I said. Older women. Let's think about why. Why is it a little creepy when an older woman wants a younger man and it's just fine when an older man wants a younger woman?

It's squirmy, said Paula. Because women get squirmy— like the chin wattle. Or those little skin flaps you get under your arms.

I don't get them there. On my neck.

Wherever. Plus the teeth—

No! I said. I do not want to talk about teeth.

You know those Museum School students who work for Ettore? Sometimes I look at their gums—their *gums*—and I envy them. Paula sighed.

I know. Their nice pink healthy gums. I rolled my leaf and put it in the pot. We're not getting anywhere. Fifty-year-old men can have nasty gums too. We haven't explained it.

It's all about babies. They want those rosy cheeks and those full pouty lips and those yummy breasts—she was

hetting and squeezing her breasts as she talked—and everything that says, Yum yum, fucky fucky, baby baby.

I *know!* I said. I know why the men want the young
women.

But that's why they don't want us, see? said Paula.

I get it, for God's sake. But why do the young women
want the old men? It isn't fair.

Fair. Ffffft.

Colette married her stepson, I said. At least, I think she
did.

Colette wore lipstick.

How do you know?

Done, she said. She rolled up the last leaf.

We ladled on the sauce and put the pot in the oven to
cook.

Oh Paula, I said. I put my head down on the table. Is it
really all over? Would it be just as all over if my vagina still
worked?

Who's to say? said Paula.

You're being diplomatic, I said, raising my head. That's
unlike you.

Accentuate the positive, said Paula. Eliminate the nega-
tive.

Let's call the whole thing off, I said.

That's a different song. You say tomayto. Don't mess
with Mister In-between. That's the next line.

Don't mess with Mister Anybody is more like it, I said.

A Dream

I woke at three or four—too dark to read the clock. It was my boyfriend. He was back. Nothing in particular happened. It was just the intensity of his desire, the perpetual, unsatisfiable wanting to fuck me. Everywhere I looked or went, he was there unzipping his pants. If we did it in the morning, he wanted to do it again after lunch, and after dinner too.

In the dream I looked out on a wasteland of desire. The landscape was cold and dry, and its only features were fucking and fucking. I could find no escape.

I shook myself awake enough to dispel the dream. And I managed to fall back asleep. When I woke up again, I was puzzled. My boyfriend had moved out more than a year before: Why was I dreaming of him now?

I wasn't surprised that my vagina hurt for several days afterward.

But it wasn't about him. It was about the aridity of my desire. I was the one who couldn't be satisfied, whose idea of love was sexual conquest. My boyfriend was crude, but he'd managed to stay focused on me. I couldn't sustain interest. I liked excitement. I always wanted a new passion to replace the one that had fizzled out. And that was my wasteland, from which I could find no escape.

Except I'd found one. My sore vagina.

But now I didn't need it, because my sexual allure, on which I'd traded for most of my life, was fading away.

Gynecology

It was time for my annual gynecological checkup.

Things must be better, said Doctor Tony. I haven't seen you in a while.

About a year, I said. Things are better than they were.

So tell me, he said.

The pain is intermittent, I said. Sometimes I have a week or two with no pain. And when it gets irritated, it settles down again pretty quickly, a couple of days.

What things irritate it? he asked.

Taking a bath, I said. A shower is okay, but it hates sitting in hot water. Too much driving—it hates that.

And how about intercourse?

I can't find anyone to try with, I said.

Doctor Tony grinned as if he didn't believe me.

It's not funny, I told him. It's true.

Okay, he said. Let me have a look.

We got the sheet arranged and he looked inside.

All normal, all fine, he said. He poked here and there. And those red spots are gone.

The one inside, I said. But there's still this one up near the clitoris.

He poked there too.

Ow, I said.

Sorry, said Doctor Tony. That spot is smaller, though, and less red. He pulled out the speculum and pushed his little rolling stool aside.

Now it's stinging and stinging, I said.

When you agitate the nerve fibers, they can't stop firing, he said.

That doesn't augur well for my sex life, if it has a fit from a speculum, I said.

Doctor Tony raised his eyebrows. Who knows, he said. A speculum isn't very exciting.

I laughed. Listen, I said, is this a neurological problem? It's as if my vagina can't process sensation correctly. As if any sensation feels like pain.

That's just what's wrong with it, he said.

Shouldn't I go to a neurologist? I asked.

I've sent some patients with this to neurologists, and they send them right back. They think it's gynecological.

Well, it's both, isn't it? I asked.

Yes, he said, it is both.

You have other patients with this? I asked him.

Some, he said. Then he said, Maybe you should try acupuncture.

Acupuncture! No, I said. I did all that stuff. I sat in baking soda and tea bags, and none of it did a thing for me.

Acupuncture can work, said Doctor Tony.

It works if you believe in it, I said. Placebo effect.

I think it's a real effect, he said. Down the hall—he waved his hand toward the other doctors' offices—at the incontinence clinic, they're sending some patients to acupuncture. Listen, one needle in the ankle and these women aren't incontinent anymore. Cured!

So how does it work? I asked.

Nerve pathways, he said. Something.

Something, I repeated. But what? And is it going to work for this? I pointed at my crotch.

It's worth a try, he said.

I didn't say anything for a minute.

Then I said, But why did I get it in the first place?

Ah, said Doctor Tony softly.

D on't separate the mind from the body. Don't separate even character—you can't. Our unit of existence is a body, a physical, tangible, sensate entity
with perceptions and reactions that express it and form it
simultaneously.

Disease is one of our languages. Doctors understand
what disease has to say about itself. It's up to the person
with the disease to understand what the disease has to say
to her.

My vagina keeps trying to get my attention. It has
something important to say to me. I'm listening.

I'm still listening.

Printed in the United States
by Baker & Taylor Publisher Services